Art as a Language for Au

Art as a Language for Autism addresses the clinical challenges that are common in working with autistic spectrum disorder by exploring how artistic expression can provide a communicative language for younger clients who are set in their thought processes and preferences.

Exploring how both art and play-based approaches can be effective tools for engaging therapeutic work, this book introduces strategies to help young clients find expressive "languages" that can fully support communication, expression, and empathic understanding, as well as build skills for relaxation, calming, and coping. Building from a foundation of a client's individual strengths and interests, this playful and integrative approach is informed by an awareness of the individual sensory profiles and the developmental needs of children and adolescents with autism. Through a greater awareness of these materials and processes for therapy, the reader will be able to create a space for their young clients to share what they know and care about.

This exciting new book is essential reading for clinicians working with children and adolescents on the autism spectrum.

Jane Ferris Richardson is an art therapist, an exhibiting artist, a play therapist, and an associate professor of art therapy at Lesley University. Her developmentally based, integrative approach to working with children merges both art and play.

"Working in the dance space I have found that when we make assumptions about a child's ability to develop and communicate, we only place limitations on the child that are based on a very narrow understanding of them until *they* reveal themselves to us. *Art as a Language for Autism* is the most wonderful and welcome addition to this perspective which provides the reader with insights of a powerful creative approach to building relationships and reimagining life changing outcomes for children and their families. Written with decades of hands-on clinical experience and a rich in-depth academic knowledge of art and play based therapeutic practice, Jane's work is truly ground-breaking and offers inspiring pathways to following and discovering the potential within each unique child."

—**Ali Golding, MSc, PG Cert SEN, BA(Hons), FRSA**,
Founder, Director, Artistic Director of MovementWorks

"In this much-needed contribution to the lexicon of ASD literature, Dr. Richardson informs clinicians, educators, and parents on the value of creative approach with children on the spectrum. Richardson frames art as a means of communication for a population that typically struggles with this; indeed, she reminds us that art is fundamental expression. The words and experiences of her young clients are shared with a genuine respect, and Richardson anchors these anecdotes by expertly weaving in the theory of art and play therapists, psychologists, and autism researchers. I look forward to recommending this text to students, clients, and colleagues."

—**Dr. Rachel Brandoff, Ph.D., ATR-BC, ATCS, LCAT**,
Assistant Professor & Coordinator of Art Therapy Concentration, Community & Trauma Counseling Program, Thomas Jefferson University

"This thoughtful book weaves links between the Reggio Emilia humanistic approach and art therapy. The Italian educational philosophy perceives a child as competent, whole, and part of society. Jane Ferris Richardson adapted it in-depth into the world of art therapy and autism in particular. Through a prolific kaleidoscope of stories, she demonstrates processes adjusted precisely to each individual. She playfully combines many nonverbal communicational languages: visual arts, music, movement, play, sand tray, storytelling, in a profound attunement to each client. The scope of interventions is rich and integrates the connections between mind, brain, and senses. She demonstrates how the arts are crucial in therapy and sometimes the only way to approach a person, especially with children with autism. This book is a meaningful contribution to those interested in art therapy, play therapy and intend to work with people with autism."

—**Nona Orbach**, *a multidisciplinary artist, therapist, blogger, presenter. Latest book:* The Good Enough Studio

"Jane Ferris Richardson has created a powerful and intriguing look at working with autistic children in her book *Art as a Language for Autism: Building Therapeutic Relationships with Children and Adolescents on the Autism Spectrum*. Richardson has skillfully interwoven the intersection of the therapeutic powers of play with the healing components of art and expressive intervention. This book presents client examples, research support, and art and play interventions throughout. Among the highlights is a chapter dedicated to adolescents and a chapter portraying a powerful illustration of a mother and son and their journey/connection through art. This book will speak to the creative and expressive therapists who work with autistic children and their families. It is also a powerful read and insight for parents and families. The power and relevance of art with autistic individuals has been lacking in literature. Richardson does an excellent job of negating this oversight."

—**Dr. Robert Jason Grant**, *creator of AutPlay® Therapy*

Art as a Language for Autism

Building Effective Therapeutic Relationships With Children and Adolescents

Jane Ferris Richardson

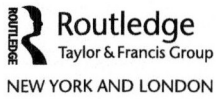
Routledge
Taylor & Francis Group
NEW YORK AND LONDON

Cover art by Gabriel Richardson

First published 2022
by Routledge
605 Third Avenue, New York, NY 10158

and by Routledge
4 Park Square, Milton Park, Abingdon, Oxon, OX14 4RN

Routledge is an imprint of the Taylor & Francis Group, an informa business

© 2023 Taylor & Francis

The right of Jane Ferris Richardson to be identified as author of this work has been asserted in accordance with sections 77 and 78 of the Copyright, Designs and Patents Act 1988.

All rights reserved. No part of this book may be reprinted or reproduced or utilised in any form or by any electronic, mechanical, or other means, now known or hereafter invented, including photocopying and recording, or in any information storage or retrieval system, without permission in writing from the publishers.

Trademark notice: Product or corporate names may be trademarks or registered trademarks, and are used only for identification and explanation without intent to infringe.

Library of Congress Cataloging-in-Publication Data
A catalog record for this title has been requested

ISBN: 978-1-138-04304-6 (hbk)
ISBN: 978-1-138-04305-3 (pbk)
ISBN: 978-1-315-17330-6 (ebk)

DOI: 10.4324/9781315173306

Typeset in Times New Roman
by Apex CoVantage, LLC

This book is dedicated to the memory of Joanne Lara, dancer, teacher, author, and the originator of Autism Movement Therapy, who reminded me that, "children show us who they are through their art."

Contents

Foreword By Shaun McNiff   ix
Acknowledgments   xii

1 Introduction: The Rainbow Day   1

2 Listening to What We May Not Hear   15

3 A Strong Image of the Child With Autism   28

4 Finding a Language for Feeling   36

5 Who Is Diagnosis For?   45

6 A World Between Art and Play   57

7 Playful Art and Artful Play: An Integrative Approach to Art and Play in Therapy   70

8 Trusting the Process in Autism   93

9 Clay, Play, and Connection   98

10 From Perfectionism to Playfulness   108

11 Empathy: Understanding the Other Through Art and Play   117

12 Potential and Possibility for Adolescents   125

13 The Spectrum and the Continuum   142

14 Experience Becomes a Doorway: A Parent's Story:
    Based on Interviews With Jennifer Damian   163

15 Conclusion   171

    References   179
    Index   191

Foreword

By Shaun McNiff

For five decades I have exhorted colleagues to approach all forms of artistic expression as integral to one another while doing the same with therapy and education, recognizing the need to support the infinitely unique ways that we learn and engage the world. Jane Ferris Richardson addresses these questions and advances an integrative vision of art and experience with depth, consummate artistry, and compelling practicality—all presented with clear, direct language. She fuses the disciplines of education and therapy, cognition and emotion, together with all forms of artistic expression, in making the case for imaginative learning environments designed to further community through the engagement of the various needs and strengths of individual persons. The creative approaches to engaging others presented in this book can serve as a model for not only dealing with the specific conditions of autism but more comprehensive professional practice in therapy and education.

Common sense tells us that children and adolescents will benefit from personalized approaches to learning designed in response to the different paths that each of us creates to hopefully attain shared human goals and competencies. Yet the structures of our professions and institutions tend to go contrary to nature, creating silos and arbitrary divisions between facets of experience that hinder generative interdependence. I keep asking, is it possible for therapy and education to realize the fullness and creative reciprocity we hope to further in life?

Helping young people learn and grow is a humbling process since we can never assume that what may work today, or in the past, will be effective tomorrow. With art, and unlike science, we do not exactly replicate procedures nor precisely predict the end at the beginning. Teaching and therapy, as well as raising our children, are creative disciplines that require commitment to relationship building and experimentation. Uncertainty in the creative process is the norm. The same goes for inevitable setbacks, all demanding the ability to stay committed, trusting that there is an intelligence at work within the complex of creation that tends to move a few steps ahead of the reasoning mind which reflects upon, appreciates, and incorporates what emerges beyond its controls (McNiff, 1998).

Problems, and especially acute difficulties, invariably stimulate us to try something different and new. Effectiveness in my experience is proportionate to the ability to respond and embrace what occurs outside the lines of expectation and do our best to support others in the process of creating their distinctive lives. Rather than assuming we, or our professions, know the way, we assist children and adolescents in finding their paths through the complex of experience that we all face. The methods of practice are in many ways antithetical to a more general desire for predictability, control, and replicable outcomes that permeate contemporary life. It might be helpful in deepening our empathy for people living with autism to reflect on how qualities of the condition such as the reluctance to change, and strict adherence to repeated behaviors, more subtly permeate life in general. The young people of this book are our teachers and guides as we are hopefully theirs.

Jane Ferris Richardson offers a depth and variety of vignettes demonstrating how her work with children and adolescents living with autism responds to the one-of-a-kind nature of each situation where disciplines of practice converge their resources in response to the needs of the moment. Rather than the application of stock methods too often seen today in therapy and education, each engagement is co-created. Notwithstanding the roles and responsibilities of those who offer professional services, the experience is permeated by mutual creation where improvisation and ongoing decision-making characterize an overall process that tends to involve feeling our way toward goals and well-being.

For example, since autism tends to seriously limit spoken language, this book explores the creation of a "multi-sensory" artistic "language to explore emotions and experiences" which also supports the enhancement of "verbal communication." In dealing with autism, where our usual modes of relating to one another and the world may be unavailable, we must create alternatives. Invariably, what works in a particular therapeutic context can be extended to life as a whole. Necessity helps us to do what we might not otherwise consider. The resulting processes correspond to what K. K. Gallas describes in using all forms of artistic expression as "languages of learning" with young children in classroom communities (1991, 1994) and Edith Cobb's exploration of how the "ecology of imagination in childhood" is the basis for lifelong creation (1992).

Jane Ferris Richardson makes important contributions to this tradition with her exploration of creativity and learning occurring within the challenging context of autism and its therapeutic treatment. Resistance and fears reliably accompany the positive features of creative expression in all of life. I have found it necessary to develop the capacity to stick with the struggles and discomfort as modeled in this book, to persist with trust that they are necessary elements within a larger process that requires all facets of experience. The monsters that universally appear in children's art and play (McCarthy, 2007, 2008, 2015) can serve as friends and helpers, helping us invent fresh ways of interacting with adversity. Art heals by creating with the shadows, by transforming afflictions into affirmation of life and hope for the future (McNiff, 2004, 2015). Problems are embraced as fuel for making life anew and as this book consistently documents, positive outcomes in art and play build confidence and spread to larger spheres of experience.

References

Cobb, E. (1992). *The ecology of imagination in childhood.* Spring Publications (originally published in 1977, NY: Columbia University Press).
Gallas, K. (1991). Art as epistemology: Enabling children to know what they know. *Harvard Educational Review, 61*(1), 40–50.
Gallas, K. (1994). *The languages of learning: How children talk, write, dance, draw, and sing their understanding of the world.* Teachers College Press.
McCarthy, D. (2007). *"If you turned into a monster": Transformation through play: A body-centered approach to play therapy.* Jessica Kingsley Publishers.
McCarthy, D. (Ed.). (2008). *Speaking about the unspeakable: Non-verbal methods and experiences in therapy with children.* Jessica Kingsley Publishers.
McCarthy, D. (Ed.). (2015). *Deep play.* Jessica Kingsley Publishers.
McNiff, S. (1998). *Trust the process: An artist's guide to letting go.* Shambhala Publications.
McNiff, S. (2004). *Art heals: How creativity cures the soul.* Shambhala Publications.
McNiff, S. (2015). *Imagination in action: Secrets for unleashing creative expression.* Shambhala Publications.

Acknowledgments

To the children whose artwork and stories are shared here, and to their families: you have taught me how to listen to what I may not hear, and I cannot thank you enough for enabling me to share this understanding with others.

Deep appreciation to Jennifer Damian and to Michael Tolleson Robles for their wonderful interviews and for generously sharing their time and insights.

Thanks to Krystal Demaine, Andrea Gollub, and Chunhong Wang for our shared research, cross-cultural collaboration, and the evolution of our work, from Massachusetts to Manhattan to Beijing. And to Gabryjelka Javierbieda, for tirelessly volunteering in Beijing.

To Ali Golding, Karen Howard, and Stephen Shore, for sharing travels and teaching in Delhi and Dhaka, making possible a deep investigation of expressive approaches to supporting autism. Thanks to Manish and Malvika Samnani and SOCH Gurgaon, and to Dr. Aftab Uddin, Mohammad Rafiquil Islam, and Faith Bangladesh for inviting us to share our work with professionals, parents, and children.

To Irina Katz-Mazilu and the Federation Francaise D'Art Therapeute, who invited me to explore, together with Joanne Lara, the importance of connection with nature through art and movement in a Paris master class on autism.

To Monica Wong, who encouraged the further investigation of Playful Art and Artful Play in Hong Kong at the International Art Therapy Conference: and to Stephanie Brooke and the Tokyo Expressive Therapies Conference for giving me my first opportunity to understand that the language of art for autism is indeed global.

To Shelly Goebl-Parker, for investigating along with me how Reggio inspiration informs art therapy practice, from Italy to our own classrooms and practices. And to Dorothy Garcia and Tom Harding of Art Aids Art, for understanding how art therapy practice could both be inspired by Reggio principles and support early childhood learning; and for inviting my students and me to Khayelitsha.

To the Expressive Therapies Summit for believing that expressive approaches are "better together," and for providing so many opportunities to collaborate with other therapists and artists. Thanks to Elaine Hall and Kerry Bowers for being among this group of colleagues.

To Debra Muzikar of The Art of Autism for the wonderful resources and insight she has so generously shared.

And much appreciation to everyone who read the chapters in progress: Nancy Jo Cardillo for discussions of empathy, Helen Cassidy Page for her reflections on sand tray, Connie Gretsch of Art Therapists for Human Rights for her understanding of how a strong image of the child supports the rights of children with autism, Shawn McGivern, for her integrative grasp of an integrative approach, Amy O'Donnell and Ron Fortier for sharing their respective artists' feedback on the Expressive Therapies Continuum, and Kathy Westgate Vena for her understanding of Reggio "languages," both as a fellow parent and as a therapist. Thanks to Nona Orbach for sharing her Reggio informed perspective on materials for art therapy.

The editorial support of Isabel Crabtree and Alex Kaptitan helped to move the book forward; and Amanda Devine, Grace McDonell, and Katya Porter at Routledge supported this work with great patience. My Lesley colleagues Lauren Leone and Andre Ruesch provided invaluable advice from their experience as authors.

Finally, to my own family, many, many thanks for your patience with the long process of researching and writing this book. Thanks to David Richardson for his careful reading of both text and photos; and for lending his trained eye to help tell children's stories visually. And thanks to Gabriel Richardson, both for his generosity in allowing the use of his artwork on the cover, and for his understanding of my work from his perspective as an artist.

The writing of this book was supported in part by sabbatical funds and through faculty development grant funding from Lesley University.

Chapter 1

Introduction
The Rainbow Day

"Is this your favorite thing? When kids come to see you here and you get to make things?" A child asked me this question as he put the finishing touches on a boat he was constructing from paper, getting ready to float it across the water filling my sand tray. To understand children's lives and worlds, therapists must listen to what they may not hear, learning about what helps a child to feel safe, and about what is important to them. Autistic children's and adolescents' special interests can be an important part of how they introduce themselves to others, coming in to a therapy session with stuffed animals, action figures, or a pocket stuffed with rocks, and connecting right away to the objects in the environment that resonate with these interests.

For a child, this may mean gravitating to the shelves of figures for play in the sand, often echoing what they have already shared through drawing.

Asking children "what is interesting to you?" and "what do you care about?" is one way to learn about what motivates and moves them; and the answer need not be in words. Yet the question is serious. With adults I suggest that they consider what is interesting to them, and that they draw a picture of something they care about when I give a workshop on art and play therapy. The first time I used this approach, I received a drawing of a steer from Temple Grandin, who was the keynote presenter for the conference, sitting in on my workshop. This interest motivated her life's work.

Through art, play, and the therapeutic relationship, children's intentions, as well as their imagination, can be supported. Helping children to communicate their own intentions and interests engages them in the process of therapy. One child with an extraordinary ability to create moveable, magical creatures, came into my room for the first time holding a flying beast he had made entirely out of paper.

This creature explored the room with him, perching on the doll's house, and looking down at the shelves full of art materials and the objects used for play in the sand tray. When the child was ready, he sat and created a beautifully articulated figure from clay, sharing not only the story of his creation, but also the story of his challenging day at school. We appreciated his strengths, and then thought together about what was difficult for him

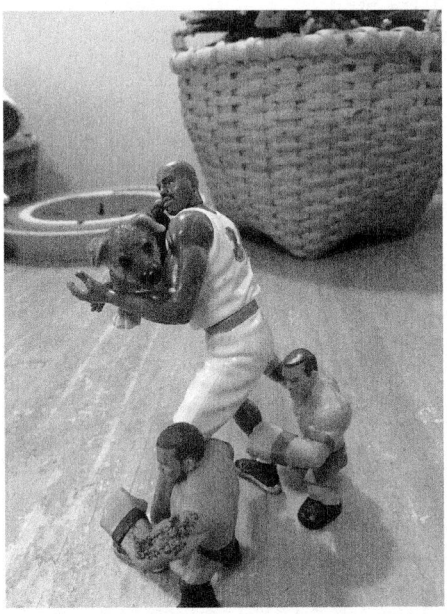

Figure 1.1 Special interests as found on the sandtray shelves.

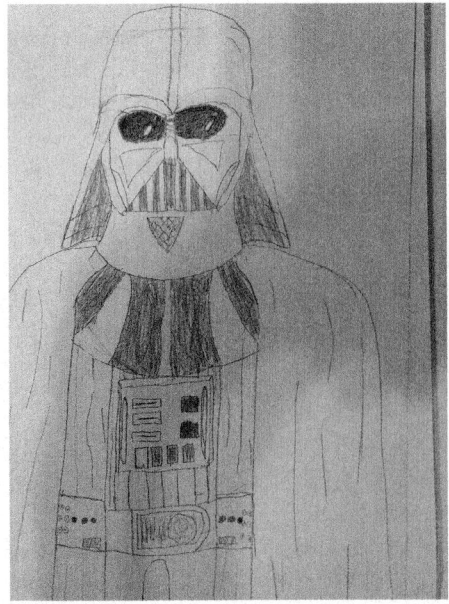

Figure 1.2 Portrait of Darth Vader by an adolescent with a special interest in Star Wars.

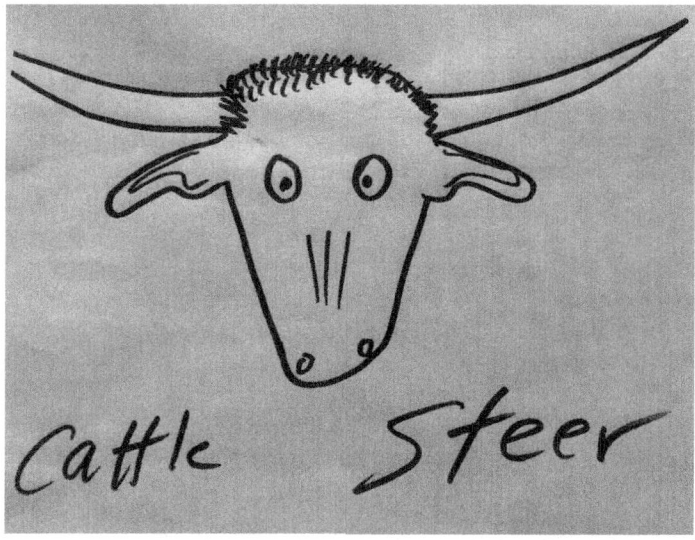

Figure 1.3 Temple Grandin's portrait of a steer, drawn in response to the author's request to draw, "something you are really interested in, something you really care about." Courtesy of Temple Grandin.

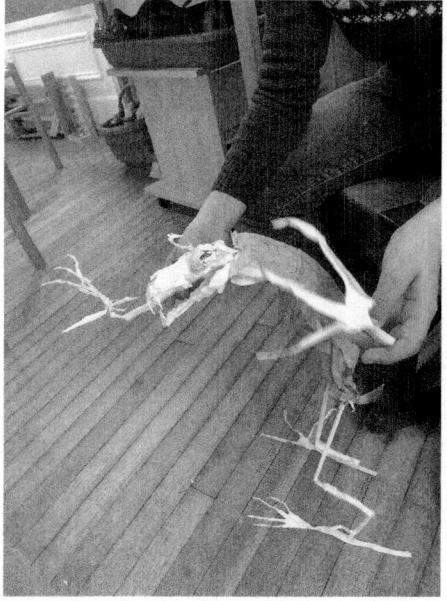

Figure 1.4 The flying creature.

and what he would like to change. These strengths become more visible and these challenges can become more manageable when they are shared and seen in perspective.

What children or adolescents themselves consider significant and respond to through art or in play is deeply connected to their interests, their approach to the world, and their areas of comfort or discomfort. Helping them to find, and communicate through, their own "language" is a task which demands flexibility from the therapist, especially with children and adolescents who can be, by virtue of their neurological makeup, inflexible. The support we give for the many ways of communicating can strengthen relationships, enhance expression, and allow for the discovery of strengths. During a game of catch, a child and I each named something we liked when we caught the ball. I was coached by the excited child to respond with "Playing with me!" He then added that he too liked to come and play, and to make art together.

Children show us who they are through their art, as Joanne Lara, the founder of Autism Movement Therapy has often observed (personal communication, April 1, 2019). Sharing their art enables others to know a child more fully. As one child explained, when you have an idea, "you can think of it . . . you can even draw it . . . and THEN you can talk about it." For him, drawing was both a comfortable way to share, in his words, "something that is new," and a way to build a relationship.

Autism impacts the mind, brain, and senses. Core challenges for children and adolescents with autism include difficulties with social communication, emotional regulation, and sensory challenges (Greenspan & Shanker, 2004; Greenspan & Wieder, 2009; Prizant et al., 2000). A holistic, individualized approach to therapy with children and adolescents with autism is based on awareness of individual needs, strengths, and challenges. The mind, brain, and senses are all engaged through making art and moving through the dynamic process of play. An integrative approach to the expressive and creative processes of art and play is flexible enough to meet the needs of children and adolescents who may have difficulty being flexible themselves; and that is the approach explored here. My training both as an art therapist and as a play therapist has been essential to developing this way of being with autistic children and adolescents, as has an understanding of individualized, developmentally based approaches to supporting different sensory needs and communication styles, and supporting emotional regulation.[1] These are resources for connecting and communicating with children and adolescents with autism in therapy and within the broader contexts of family, community, and educational settings.

Finding a language to explore emotions and experiences is essential. "Talk therapy, in particular, may not work well for autistic people, because they can struggle with social communication and with identifying their feelings"

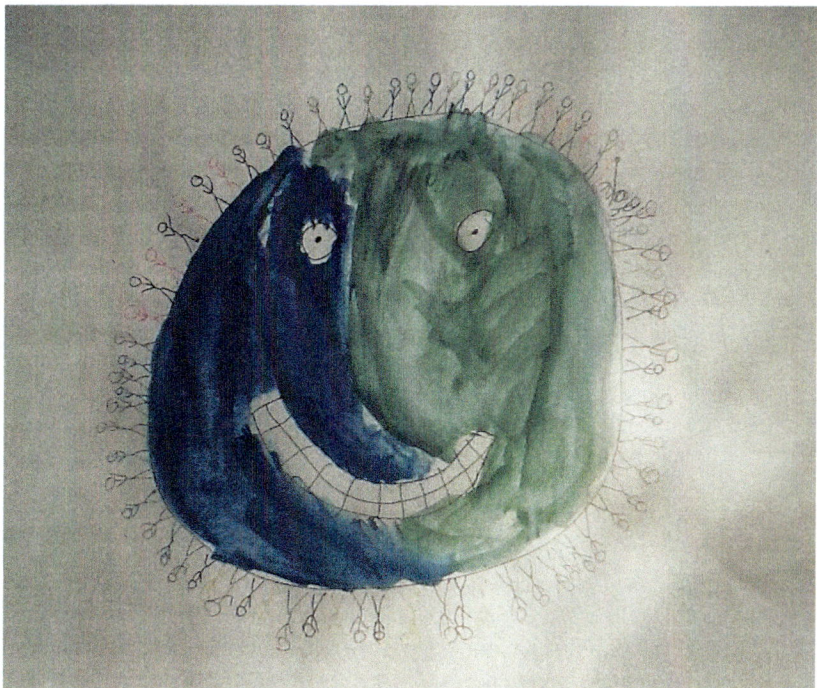

Figure 1.5 The world as a happy place.

(Weinstock, 2019). The fundamental principles of art and play based approaches rely on working with the nonverbal but richly expressive languages of art, and the process of play. Play and art, as the Reggio educators understand, "are experiences and explorations of life, of the senses, and of meanings" (Gandini et al., 2005, p. 9). Supporting children to trust in the process of play and art making allows for this exploration. In the words of one young girl I saw in therapy, therapists help children to experience and represent the world as "a friendly place, most of the time."

When I see children and adolescents with autism in individual therapy, the goals for our work together may include navigating difficult transitions at school or in the family, or helping to manage anxiety or feelings of depression. Autistic children and adolescents have a higher rate of anxiety and depression. Communication, calming, and coping are important therapeutic goals to address these challenges. At the same time, it is important to explore what is possible for children and adolescents, both through holding a strong image of them and helping them to develop a sense of their own self-efficacy. The approach presented here is integrative, drawing from art and play therapy, and encompassing careful consideration of when to let a child lead, and when to offer more structure and support. The overarching goal is to better connect and communicate with children and adolescents with autism, and to support their self-expression and communication with others. In telling children's stories, I am describing "not just autistic experience, but human experience," as Raymond Foye (in Silberman & Foye, 2020) has observed of the stories of autistic people; but these experiences have autism as an integral and individual component.

As Prizant (2015) explains, "autism is called a spectrum disorder because the abilities and challenges of people with autism fall along a continuum, and no two people manifest autism in the same way" (p. 223). For diagnostic categories to be of meaningful use, both strengths and challenges must be understood in the context of an individual's life. The goal of diagnosis is to better understand each individual and to better meet their needs. The goal of therapy is not to "cure" the child or adolescent's autism. Autistic children and adolescents want to be free of their worries and anxiety. They want to be free to play, to engage with others, and to communicate. They want to be free to explore what interests and matters to them. I have found that children and adolescents often express an articulate awareness about their autism, and that, in some important ways, they do not want to be different. The language used here reflects this preference, using "autistic children," (or adolescents) and "children (or adolescents) with autism," interchangeably, to suggest how autism is both part of who the child is, and also that autism is not the entirety of who the child is.

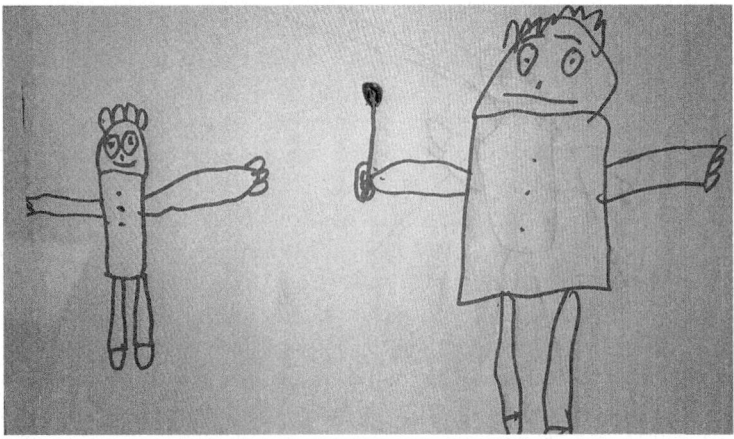

Figure 1.6 A scary dream of robbers.

Children express this awareness when they describe their experience and their goals for therapy. One fifth grader wrote in his school journal:

> I worry about people getting hurt. I worry about lots of things. I want to stop worrying some day. I hope one day. I worry about fires. I worry about robbings. I worry about accidents. I worry about bad report cards. I worry about people. People getting beat up. And I worry about the pets.

And yet, when he reflected on his autism, he shared his sense that "autism is a special thing," and a part of him which helps him to do certain things better. He explained that:

> I can't touch my autism because it's inside me . . . autism is a special thing . . . most people don't get . . . most people don't HAVE it so they can't understand. You can't feel it or touch it because it's inside . . . people who have it don't act like a normal person. Sometimes people with autism are really good at music . . . they're smart and good at things.

And a teen girl explained that "I don't want to be so different . . . and change what I like to do . . . I DO want to have friends . . . I want people to understand what I need . . . to feel comfortable."

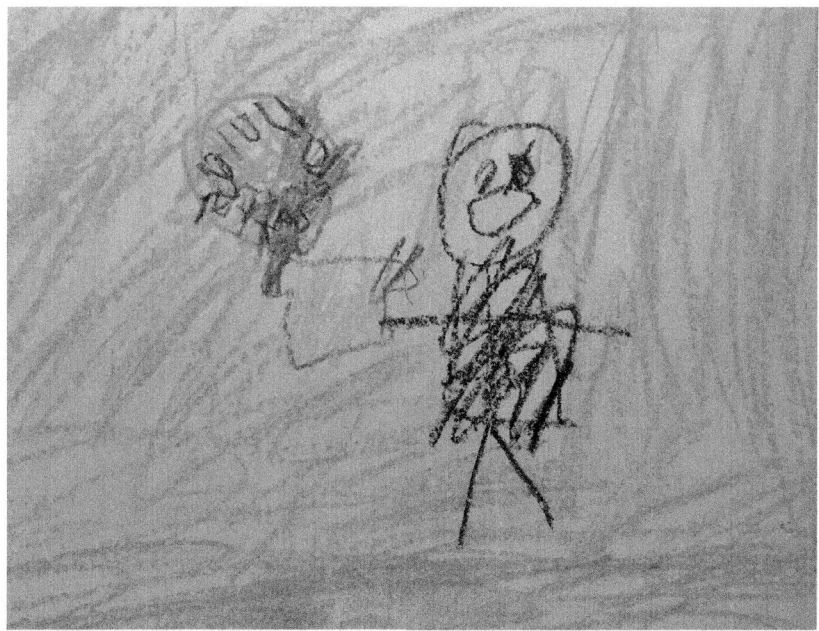

Figure 1.7 Portrait of the author with a snack—a piece of home baked toast—prepared by a child.

In the process of building comfort in the therapy setting, children and adolescents connect with the environment and materials as well as with the therapist.

The inherently calming effects of drawing, painting, or shaping clay can be soothing and self-regulating. Working with responsive and flexible materials can encourage flexibility in the child or adolescent. There is a huge difference, for example, between how it feels to work with flowing paint and with more contained crayons or pencils. All children or adolescents will certainly not be attracted to or choose to explore all materials. Exploration of new materials and processes, however, can lead to increased flexibility and new insights.

When I met a young child in my waiting room one day, he was wearing special rainbow glasses. He encouraged me to look through them at the chandelier hanging in the hallway, which did indeed look unusually brilliant and shimmering. What a wonderful invitation this was from a child to experience my familiar world in a different way. As we moved into the art and play room, he took out a rainbow xylophone, playing music that made him feel "relaxed and happy," and saying, "this is how I warm up." We had shared the idea of getting comfortable and warming up by moving, doing something active to feel comfortable following a long day of school.

As the tones of the xylophone faded he announced, "we're going to have a rainbow day." He had carefully observed the room, and told me, "you really like rainbows," because I have so many colorful play materials, and so many colors and ranges of paint. We had experimented with a relaxation story that takes a child through the colors of the rainbow, a process he had enjoyed and returned to again and again. Relaxation, explains Khalsa (2016), like other structured but comforting experiences, can be successful when therapists see what children are interested in and connect with these interests (p. 122) in a way that supports the need for regulation. Siegel (2012) explains how, "the flow of energy and information from the body up into the cortex changes our bodily states, our emotional states, and our thoughts" (p. 59). Our playful engagement with rainbows had provided this regulation for him, and now he was exploring how to create comfort for himself.

We agreed that we both liked rainbows, recollecting his painting and clay work depicting rainbows, a theme he had returned to several times. While I always try to connect with children through their own special interests and sensory preferences, here he was also noticing and thinking about my interests, and what interests we shared. This child especially loved my basket of minerals and collection of crystals and geodes, and sometimes he brought in rocks and minerals from his own collection to show me. As Courtney (2017) has suggested, "when children see the objects of nature in the office, they want to reach out and touch them. It is not enough to look with the eye—they are connecting to an inner primordial urge to know their world through engaged contact" (p. 107).

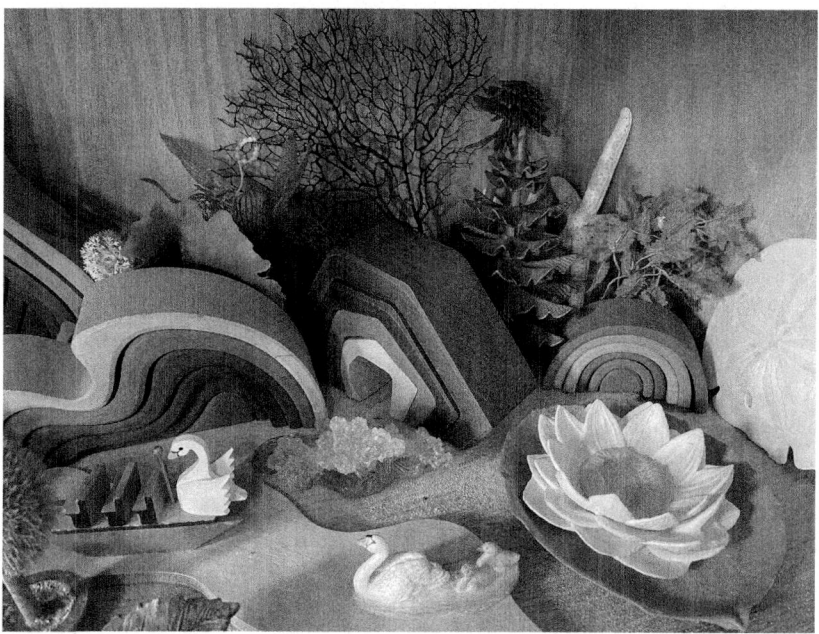

Figure 1.8 Sandtray shelf with images of nature and natural materials.

While we talked about rainbows, we experimented with the prisms from my basket of fidgets, each of us moving the light they reflected around the room in a shared dance. He then decided to put a large wooden rainbow in the sand tray. We devised a way to take a picture of his perspective on this sandtray world together.

While he held the prismatic glasses, I aimed my camera through the glasses and into the sand. He decided that everything would be upside down in this sandtray world, and that the rule here would be, "no right side up people."

He was seeing, and helping me to see, things from a different perspective. Through the construction of the world the child builds in the sand, the therapist is literally introduced to their point of view in a dynamic and evolving way. As he began to choose buildings and people to inhabit his world, I made careful notes of his actions and words, following his play and the emergence of his thoughts about the scene he was creating. My task here was to help him feel connected to his play, so that he could fully experience, and then share, his story (Richardson, 2012). He felt comfortable enough to grab a pen, and add his own rule about no "right side up people" to my written narrative of his play. He then grabbed a smiling stress ball and said "now it's a frown," but added that people were happy to be in the world, and that there was nothing "creepy"

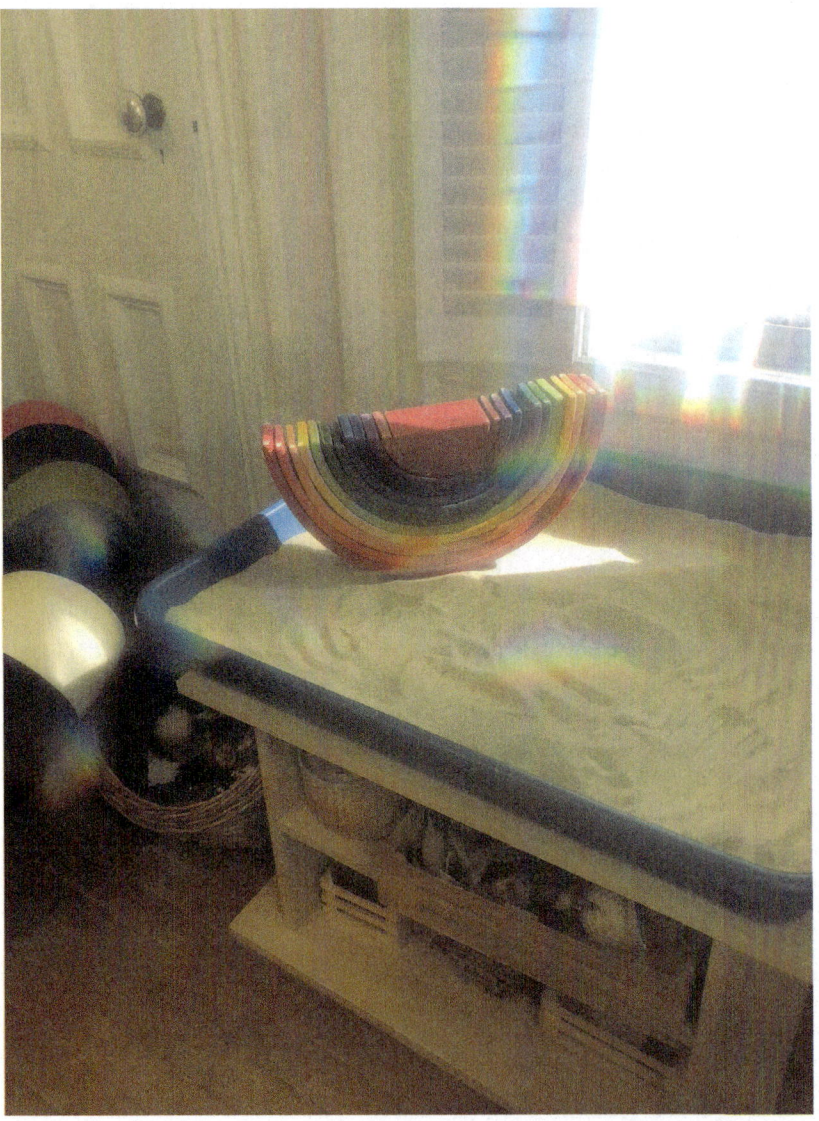

Figure 1.9 The sand tray photographed with a child through their prismatic glasses.

Introduction 11

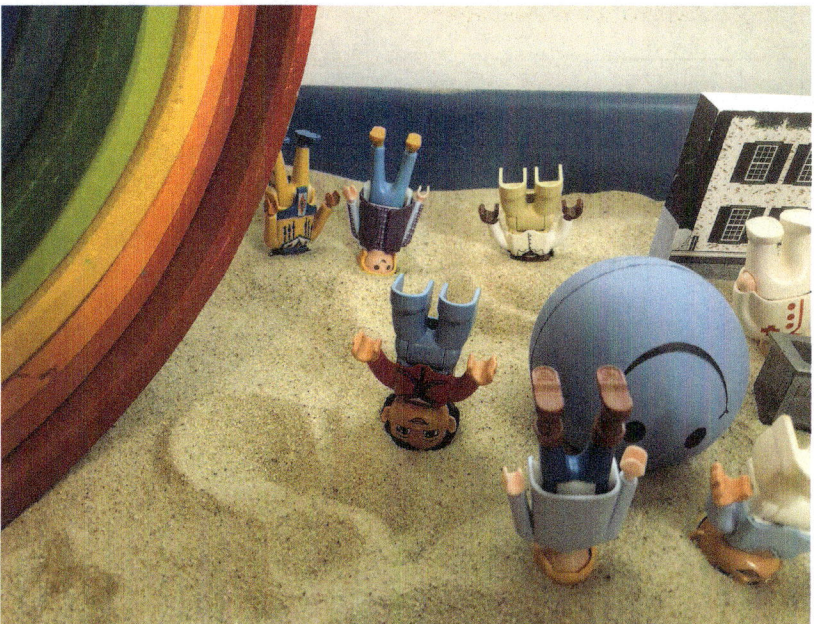

Figure 1.10 The upside down world in the sand tray.

there. This detail was very important, as he had been struggling with persistent fears that were amplified by his vivid imagination. The story of this child, and the other stories of children and adolescents shared here, are told from the perspective of a "strong image" of the child, inclusive of their strengths as well as their challenges. Common themes are explored through stories which may draw from more than one child's experience in therapy; but the developmental stages of children and adolescents are carefully delineated. Particular attention has been paid to the ways in which children and adolescents with autism creatively use the arts and play to enhance calming, coping, and communication. The growth of relationship and empathic understanding is an important component of this therapeutic process.

While the therapist serves as a witness to the child's play, observing and noting the direction of the play, children may invite the therapist to actively join in their play, as this child did on this day. Such an invitation can help the child bring their play to life, and to engage and communicate more fully with the therapist. We experimented with looking at his peaceful world by turning upside down ourselves, looking through our legs at the sand tray. We talked about how that was a bit harder to do than looking right side up, but

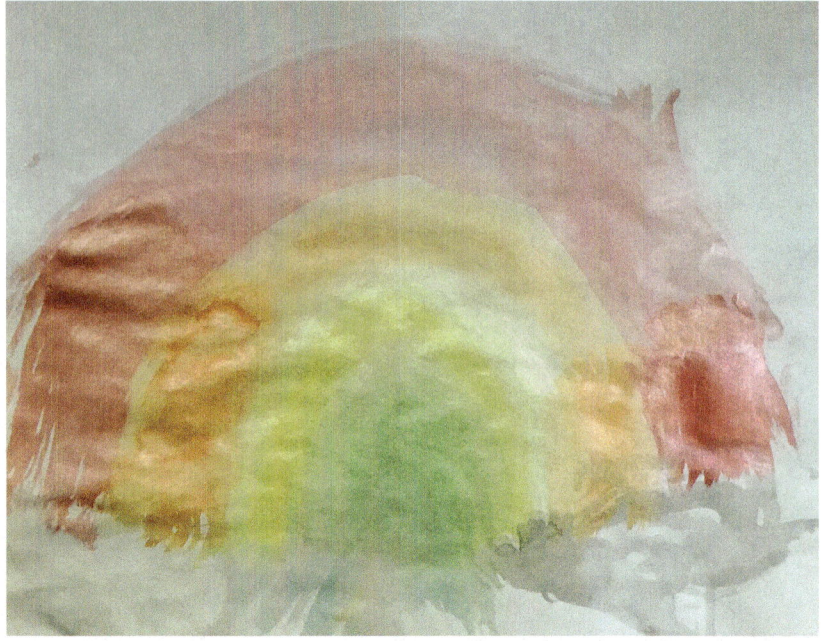

Figure 1.11 The painted rainbow supported by clouds.

"interesting and fun." I shared that I was happy to see his world the way he had created it, and how special it was to look through his rainbow glasses.

The sand tray is a place where ideas, emotions, and fascinations become visible (Richardson, 2012). I was interested as well to see the way in which he moved both into, and out of, playing in the sand during this session, which offered so many moments of shared play, art making, and communication. When he finished with his sand tray, he decided he wanted to "throw up the rainbow," using silk scarves in sensory play. We took turns throwing a big pile of colorful silk scarves and letting them land on top of us. With time remaining, I asked if he would like to paint a rainbow, so that he could have this image to keep. He chose the pearlescent paints to give the shimmering color that we saw through his glasses.

He said, "I always like to paint the clouds," and carefully added them. This gave us another opportunity to look back on what we had done together, both on this day, and also over the course of our time together. Rainbows were a theme that recurred in his art and play. In sharing his play, I was able to acknowledge the significance of these particular images, and the themes that he had expressed in his play. He too was able to experience satisfaction with his sense of focus and mastery, but also to enjoy the playfulness and relaxation of our time together. As De Domenico has said of Sandtray Worldplay, "When we enter into our creations, we explore ourselves" (personal communication, August 5, 2004). His creations helped us both to see beyond his challenges to his growth.

This session incorporated music, movement, and sandtray play, as well as painting and creating digital imagery. He moved between different languages. He alternated between play that he initiated, and receptivity to suggestions from me as the therapist. He both shared and invited me to take his perspective. I had the opportunity to see as he sees through his special glasses, both right side up, and upside down. Together we looked into the world of the sand tray and at his flowing painting. He had been working on mastery of fears, finding comfort in social settings, and regulation of affect. He accessed all the tools we had been exploring in therapy, finding regulation and communicating his needs. This session, and this imagery, served as a sort of touchstone in the therapy process.

In later sessions we revisited and built on things he had done on this very active day. When he was feeling stressed and frustrated, he searched through my materials and found bubble wrap. His face brightened, and he confided,

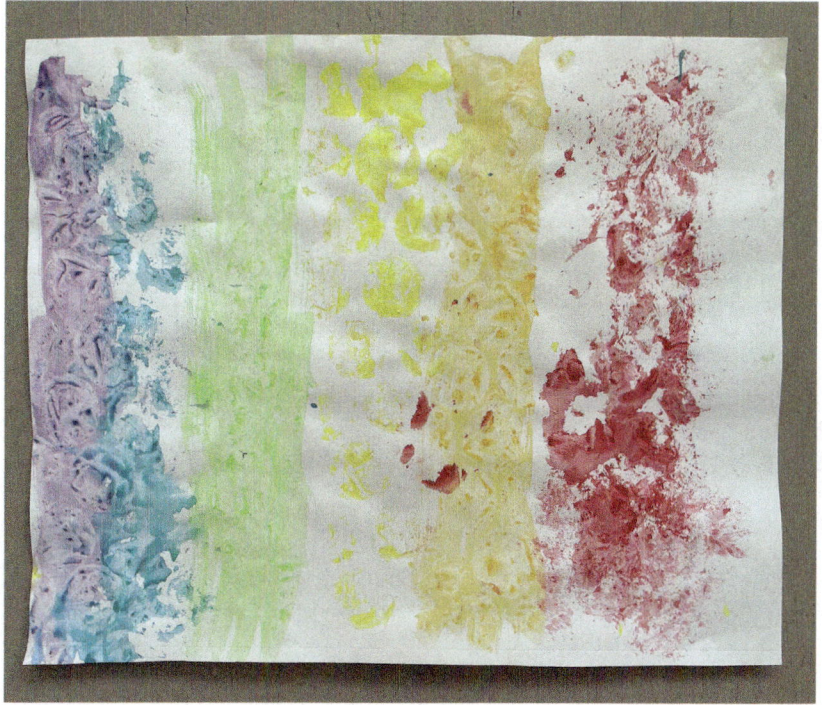

Figure 1.12 The printed rainbow.

"I love bubble wrap." I invited him to use the bubble wrap as he chose, and he wanted to pop the large bubbles. We spread it out on the floor, where pops resounded until he had flattened every last bit. When he was calmer and more relaxed, I suggested that we make something from the bubble wrap. We got out paints to make a print. He carefully began to choose the colors of the rainbow, transforming the page into a rainbow of bubbling texture and soothing color.

Children and adolescents often move not only from one form of art making to another, but also from play to art making, or from art making to play. Some children and adolescents may not respond to art materials when they first enter the therapeutic space, but they may readily communicate with the therapist through playing a drum or a xylophone, wrapping themselves in a silk scarf, or playing with puppets. "Of course," as Rubin (2005) observes, "there is a close relationship between art and play; playfulness is often part of a creative process and there is much artistry in good play therapy" (p. 350).

Communication may be clearer through the arts than it is verbally. And, in turn, the art experience may enhance verbal communication. Shore (2006a) describes how music provides structural regularity for a child with autism (p. 69), and also serves as what he terms "a carrier sign for verbal communication." Rhythm is an element in visual art making as well, and as McNiff suggests, "art can be as natural as breathing" (personal communication, March 28, 2018) when we allow rhythm to lead us into art making. Therapy offers a safe space to move into a shared rhythm with others.

Note

1 Examples of developmentally based, individualized approaches to supporting the growth of children with autism are DIR Floortime (Greenspan & Wieder, 2009), and the SCERTS method (Wetherby & Prizant, 2000). The author's training in these approaches, which includes the Floortime Basic Course and two levels of SCERTS training, has informed the broader context for this work through their emphasis on building growth-enhancing relationships. The neurologically and developmentally based approach of Autism Movement Therapy (Lara, 2016), which the author is certified to teach, has likewise been essential to understanding how the integration of the arts supports expression and individual development.

Chapter 2

Listening to What We May Not Hear

The initial communication challenge in therapy is to encourage a child to enter into the therapeutic space, and to explore what might be possible there. One day I found an adorable small girl waiting in my hallway with her earbuds firmly in her ears and a faraway expression on her face. She was willing to enter my adjoining room, invitingly full of toys and art materials, but not to take off her music player. I gestured toward her device, and gave a quizzical look, pointing towards my own ears, and wondered, as dramatically as I could, could I try hearing what she was hearing? To my initial surprise, she allowed me to do this; to literally hear part of what was going on in her head. As luck would have it, I have a large collection of puppets and animals, and was able to quickly pick out characters from her song including dancing bears, and flying horses. She watched carefully as I made them dance and fly around the room, mindful of staying just outside of her personal space. She hummed along with the song, and with me, and slowly began to explore the room. Eventually she wanted to paint, and made picture after picture filled with colors and shapes. Flowing paint led to playing the drums, and we ended together with a song that had no words but her name. This movement through space, and between materials, feels like moving between languages. It is energizing and empowering for children to make choices about how to express themselves. Children can be encouraged to see themselves as actively deciding what they would like to do in this new environment: creating, playing, and communicating. Adolescents may reflect on their relationship with the creative process. As they give a new and expressive form to the unstructured materials for art and play, their creations may feel like an expression of themselves.

In the schools of Reggio Emilia Italy (Malaguzzi, 1987), "languages" are considered to be nonverbal as well as verbal ways of expression and communication. When children are not able, or do not choose to use verbal language, then we "have to have special care for all the other languages the children CAN use" (Reggio Children, 2015). Access to many expressive languages, including the body-based languages of movement, gestures, and dance; the sound-related languages of music and speech; and the visual languages made possible by art and natural materials, expands children's understanding and their ability to communicate. Music therapist Karen Howard explains how, "we bring the invisible to the visible through the arts" (personal communication, November 29, 2018).

The processes and materials of art and play support developing expression, and the therapist's support gives children fuller access to languages for expression. Engaging autistic children through art is a means to increase flexibility, decrease perfectionism, broaden interests, and nurture talents. The therapist attunes to the child's communication, both verbal and nonverbal, to move more fully into what Prizant (in Gray, 2002) describes as "the complex dance of reciprocal social communication" (p. 4). Evans and Dubowski (2001) describe this process as, "tuning in to the children's experience as naturally and comfortably as possible" (p. 75). And Berger (2002) cautions that "interventions must make sense to the child on an emotional and a sensory level" (p. 31). For children with autism, such awareness and "tuning in" requires particular attentiveness to the child's comfort.

When combined with a flexible and playful approach, art becomes animated, and allows for movement, change, elaboration, and exchange. Sometimes children move from play to art. Sometimes they move from art to play. In a fluid transition to art making, experimentation with materials retains a playful quality for the child. Children's play and art are an invitation to experience their world together with them, mindful of seeing what may not be heard.

Support from the environment and from relationships is an essential element of encouraging art making, play, communication, and new learning. Greenspan discusses enhancing flexibility, encouraging creativity, and building meaningful communication as the fundamental therapeutic goals (Greenspan & Shanker, 2004, p. 222). However, challenges in regulating emotions can color autistic children's responses to new experiences, even in therapy. A core challenge in autism, as described by Wetherby and Prizant (2000), consists of simultaneously focusing attention and remaining responsive to others. Children who become overstimulated by this effort may understandably feel confused, becoming visibly anxious or withdrawing into self-soothing behavior. Children may also experience extreme sensitivity to environmental stimuli, whether sounds, smells, textures, or the presence of other people or particular objects. These sensory responses may be so acute and uncomfortable as to be completely distracting for a child. Henley (1992) has observed how even sharing "the same field of vision" (p. 70) while creating together can be difficult to establish.

For children whose strengths may be more visual than verbal, the mechanics, or social pragmatics, of communication may prove mystifying. Communication skills can be strengthened through art making and play, where children are able both to attend to activities and materials, and to communicate symbolically. Wetherby and Prizant (2000) describe how:

> First, with increasing capacities in joint attention children become more able to share attention, share emotions, as well as express intentions with

social partners in reciprocal interactions. Next, with increasing capacities in symbolic behavior, children develop more sophisticated and abstract means to communicate and play with others.

(p. 3)

Through play and art making, children with autism can communicate in a way that is comfortable for them. They may actively try to get inside the mind of others, starting with their therapist. One child asked me, with a serious mien, "Did you want to be a paleontologist when you were little?" This, of course, was his own dream future profession. He frequently reminded me that this might have been the case for me too, and generously advised that this profession might still be more fun than practicing art therapy, despite his considerable enjoyment of his sessions. In an act of generosity, he painted me some fossils on rocks for my sand tray. Even though he did not like to touch the sand, he knew that I loved it and thought it was important.

A young adult artist with autism, Li Jing Di, whom I met in Beijing, was able to carefully observe the presence and appearance of others. She paints sensitive portraits with traditional Chinese brush and ink. Her therapist, my close colleague Wang Chunhong, explained how they were able to "make a relationship through working together," creating art and creating connection (personal communication, August 10, 2015). Jing painted freshly and with confidence. She sensitively looked for the qualities in her subjects that she wanted to portray, gaining an understanding of others through her art.

Helping children, adolescents, and young adults to find and communicate through their own expressive "language" demands flexibility, especially with individuals who may be, by virtue of their neurological makeup, inflexible. There is a place in therapy for all the artistic and playful languages that children can embrace to support emerging abilities, expressions, and inclinations. For children with autism the communicative potential of their artwork is critically important.

Children's art offers us a unique window into the child's thoughts and feelings. Often, for children with autism, direct questioning may be acutely uncomfortable, as Frith (in Kellman, 2001) has described. But the presence of an image that has been given form in clay or taken shape on paper, offers a concrete way to communicate ideas, tell stories, or reflect on feelings. Art gives autistic children and adolescents a way to communicate with others, both through their art and about their art.

The process of making art can also help a child to articulate what is anxiety provoking for them. A child once tentatively began to talk about a bad dream. He initially said, "it's hard to talk about . . . it's too scary." He responded to the suggestion that the dream could be drawn with visible relief, and as he began to choose colors for his drawing he decided that if he could draw it, "that might be better."

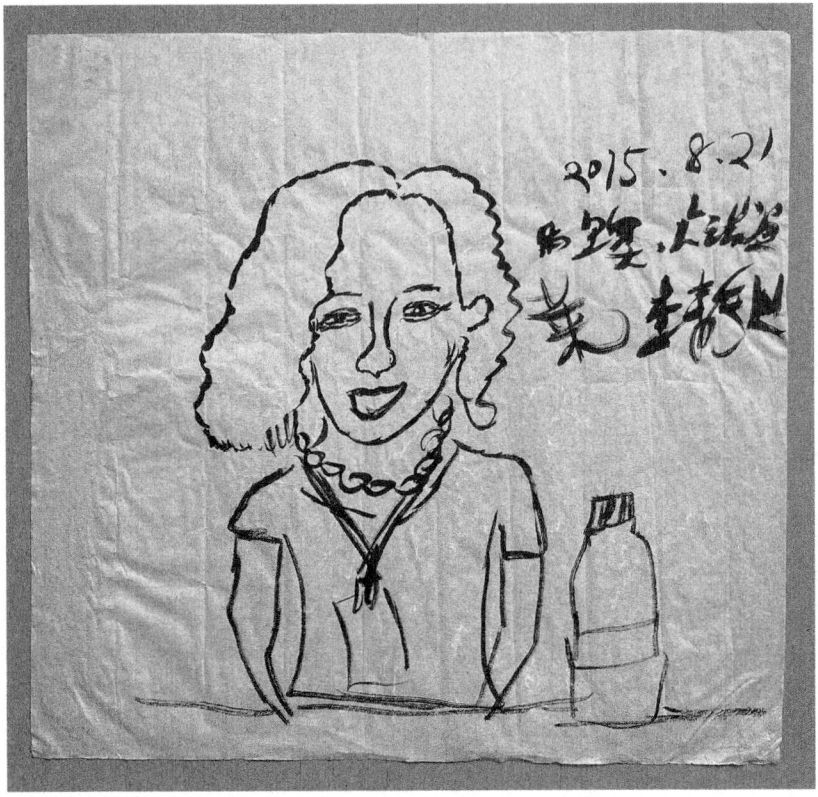

Figure 2.1 Ink portrait of the author by Li Jing Di. Collection of the author.

The artwork became a safe container for a frightening experience. Whether placing their anxiety in the sand as an image (Richardson, 2012), or their dreams on paper, children appreciate seeing the concrete depiction of their ideas and feelings, which can then be shared and looked at from a safe distance. The child who created the dream drawing confidently added his drawing to a portfolio, reminding himself that "the scary dreams go in there . . . and stay there."

Children with autism are often passionately interested in their preferred topic or activity. We can see their interest and enthusiasm come alive in art and play. Their dedication to a special interest can be extraordinary, and their sharing of these interests provides therapists with something concrete to communicate about. Special interests can bring genuine delight for children. I have seen a child literally jumping for joy out of excitement when I found a new material that piqued their interest, or doing a dance of happiness with a scarf or a shaker. The high level of interest and enthusiasm that children with autism often bring to activities that they enjoy Lovecky (2006) suggests "can be another source of creativity" (p. 222). In her study of gifted children with autism she describes the thought process in autism as "different . . . and potentially highly original" (p. 223). What children themselves consider significant is deeply connected to their interests, their approach to the world, and their areas of comfort or discomfort.

Children have arrived in my office looking listless and stating that they are "bored" without screens. When a child silently flops into a cozy seat or onto a stack of cushions, "clamming up" as Malchiodi and Crenshaw (2017) describe, finding a starting point for a session is challenging. Using sensory materials and physically exploring the room help to provide a sense of movement. One sighing child, who said he was "bored" and tired and didn't want to do anything, slowly rose from a big soft chair to pick up a large horse puppet. He gave the puppet a hug, and then began to visibly relax. He set up a "barn" for the horse, into which the child climbed as well, all the while providing blankets, food, and hugs. While the horse quietly napped, the child became increasingly animated, and clambered out of the "barn" to draw, leaving a bird puppet to watch over the horse as he slept.

While therapists, like teachers and parents, can help children to build on an area of strength and interest and to engage with others, this is only possible when we remember that, as in Temple Grandin's experience, "novelty . . . is both interesting and scary . . . it's scary if it is shoved in the face" (Grandin, 2006b). She describes how her own interests were encouraged by "the more creative types" (Grandin, 2006a) in her schools and how she brought her visual strengths into the social realm by creating costumes for school plays. In the process, she came to understand the importance of sharing an interest with others to whom it is also important.

I have often heard children talk of how the arts are an area where they can connect with others more fully, stretching their interest, much as Grandin has described. A sixteen-year-old described the theatre as "a place where I can connect." And a ten-year-old who was experiencing social challenges at school echoed how her theatre camp was the place where, "I had the most fun. I had fun because we do fun things together." Reciprocal communication comes through sharing. This outcome of shared experience may not be an easy process for children with autism, but rather is one which must be deliberately supported. Shore has emphasized the importance of helping children reframe a restricted interest into a "focused" and intentional one, where the child can both experience and share their strengths, through building self-awareness and self-esteem.

A twelve-year-old told me, "I'm good at playing the drums . . . I had fun drumming with the other kids." Another child, as he played the xylophone in my office and created music to accompany the story of his play, stopped and said, "I never knew that I was talented at music!" And, after a couple of weeks of guitar lessons, a middle school child told me, "My teacher freaked out that I already knew all those chords!"

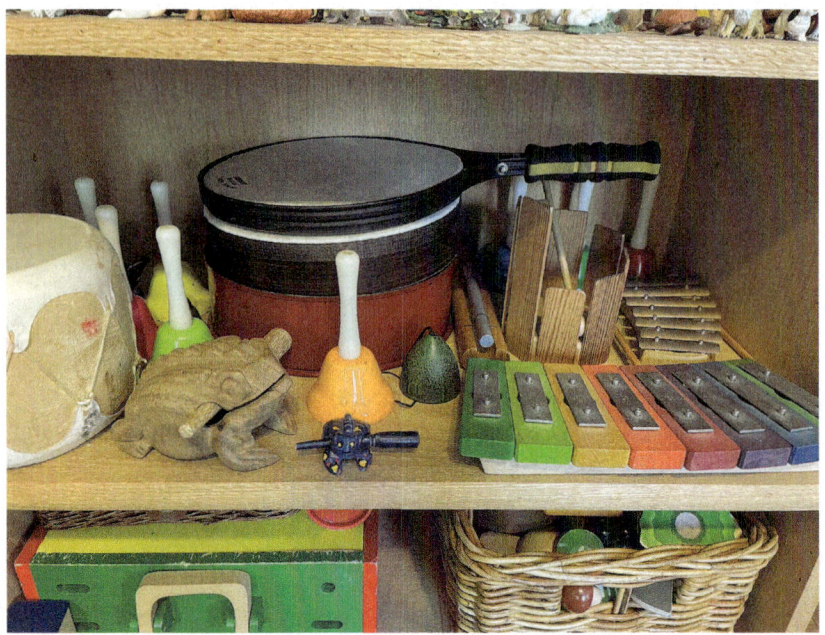

Figure 2.2 The instrument shelf with rainbow xylophone.

Shore (2006a, 2013) describes the organizing potential of music, and highlights the fact that children with autism may be very acute at hearing and possess perfect, or near perfect pitch, like the boy I was working with. Children with autism may find art, movement, or music engaging and logical in a way that fits well for them. They may display an ability to respond to music, to play an instrument, or to draw, that becomes a source of mastery as well as pleasure. Sharing through art engages us in what Moon (C. Moon, 2010) calls a relational aesthetic. From a relational perspective, the significance of art created in therapy is valued in part for "its ability to foster and deepen quality in terms of connections" (p. 142). These connections begin with a child or adolescent's connection to their own creation, and extend to both the relationship with the therapist and the developing sense of self. Ed Regensburg (2016), an art therapist who works with clients with autism, has suggested that art therapists are utilizing a different therapeutic language that innately "makes sense" to children with autism. He feels that "trust is built" when therapists use "a modality that is attuned to their frequencies" (p. 5). When children move from exploration of materials to giving a new and expressive form to these materials, their art, as Rubin (2005) says, "often feels like an extension of the self" (p. 132).

The accounts of adults with autism, who can reflect on their own experience and articulate what children cannot, offer essential guidance to therapists, educators, and parents. In contrast to Grandin's well-known description of a mind that flourishes with rich imagery, the late autistic artist and writer Donna Williams (in Richardson, 2009) spoke of an expressive process she called "artism": an interactive relationship between autism and art, which she believed worked for her on many dynamic levels. She described her own creative process as being more kinaesthetic than visual, and described how: "My mind is like a mosaic: my conscious thoughts intangible until I experience them after they've been expressed—usually through arts" (in Richardson, 2009, p. 109). Justin Canha is a young autistic artist exhibiting in New York. His parents have described how they began to help build on Justin's early interest in drawing and his visual skills to build fuller communication with him (Richardson, 2009). While they knew that they could teach Justin words and skills, it was through art that they experienced the "eureka moment" of communication with Justin. Clara Park (2001) describes her artist daughter Jessy's journey since first discovering her expressive strengths in art class. There, her mother explains, "This bizarre youngster who screamed at the bells . . . and could hardly talk, could do any assignment" (p. 23). Now, as an adult artist with a solid history of exhibitions and commissions, "art is important in itself, as autistic obsessions grow beautiful" (p. 123). And yet, there are other benefits of Jessica Park's creative work, as her mother reflects: "It brings her into contact with people. It enhances her communication skills" (p. 132), and also allows her to generate an income. For Kim Miller, art was first a means of communication, and later a source of identity and vocation. Once Kim began communicating through her art, her world widened. Her mother Eileen Miller's (2008) account *The Girl Who Spoke in Pictures* describes the growth of Kim's communication and connection through art. Miller reflected on how, "mainly because of her ability to express feelings, wants, needs and intellectual development through her art," (p. 143) Kim had a much fuller educational experience. Now, as a young woman who has gone on to illustrate children's books, she feels her creative process is essential to her life.

Children too can engage seriously with the materials and processes of artists. Kellman (2001), in her study of art making by autistic children, suggests that children and adolescents with autism often have the capacity of bringing intense focus to what they are looking at. She describes this as, "looking closely at what one wishes to draw or paint," noting that this is "one of the first and most important skills developed by an artist" (p. 46). She also found that autistic children have a propensity for looking at objects in a more sustained manner than other children. Their drawings portray "their preoccupations and purposes" (Kellman, 2001, p. 67) with great clarity. An adolescent artist with autism described working with this intent focus to me as, "releasing the image" after, "first thinking of it, and paying attention to it" (Richardson, 2009, p. 110). Younger children too can see themselves as active creators, as they move from exploring the environment and materials to creating and communicating with them.

Shore (2006a, 2006b) discusses the fundamental importance of attending to the arts as an important means of communication for children with autism. He feels that the arts provide significant resources for creating empathy, communication, and positive behavioral change. And Attwood, (in Baron et al., 2006) has described how art materials can be literal tools for relaxation, and art processes such as painting can be used to manage "uncomfortable and potentially overwhelming stressors and emotions" (p. 361). Art can bring comfort as well as expression. Shore (in Hosseini, 2012) further suggests that:

> Whether it be music, drama, visual arts, comedy, dance, or other forms of the arts, I encourage parents to "play" in creativity with their kids. While not every child will respond to every form of the arts, within every child is a connection to one form or another and a potential waiting to be fulfilled. Find your child's artistic "carrot" and you'll open a door to possibilities beyond your wildest imaginations and dreams.
> (p. 46)

This view of engaging children in art is deeply respectful of children, and assumes a strong image of children with autism.

To nurture children's strengths, the therapist must be a careful and responsive observer. Therapists look carefully at the choices children make and the images they depict with what Rubin (2005) has called a "third eye," (p. 93) or a heightened perception of both the child and the art they create. Wolfberg (2003) has suggested the importance of careful observation of the expressive play of children with autism, paying especially close attention to the symbolic dimension of play as well as to the social communication aspects of the play.

As the fit between expression and materials becomes more comfortable for children, their comfort and communication increase. Children need both the freedom to respond to new experiences and materials, and support to help them through challenges with these experiences. Henley (2018) discusses the importance of being in a shared space, where inviting materials and media can provoke a child's interest, but can also create a "buffer" for too much proximity that may feel uncomfortable to the child. This and other challenges in regulating emotions and sensory responses can color responses to new experiences, to art materials, or to the other people who present or participate in these experiences.

A significant challenge for children and adolescents with autism stems from difficulty in focusing attention while remaining responsive to others. These regulatory challenges explain the presence in my art space of balls to bounce on, large soft cushions to sit or lean on, and baskets of "fidgets" of all sorts. Sometimes, children need to circle the room, bouncing, juggling, drumming, or playing a xylophone, and interacting with me through these sensory activities.

Children may enter the therapy environment already on "overload" from their day. Sensory responses may be so acute and uncomfortable as to be completely distracting for a child. An initial challenge with children may be the difficulty of sharing the space, or even, as Henley (1992) says "sharing the same field of vision" (p. 70). Therapists work with materials and processes that hold the potential both to overwhelm and to engage children.

Art itself offers a potential focus for shared understanding and shared experience. Such shared experience is the cornerstone of children's ability for "social communication" (Wetherby & Prizant, 2000). Among the skills needed for social communication, as Wetherby and Prizant (2000) describe, are joint attention with another person and symbolic behavior:

> These two foundations of social communication underlie functional abilities in a variety of ways. First, with increasing capacities in joint attention, children become more able to share attention, share emotions, as well as express intentions with social partners in reciprocal interactions. Next, with increasing capacities in symbolic behavior children develop more sophisticated and abstract means to communicate and play with others.
>
> (p. 3)

These are skills that are greatly strengthened through play and art making. And when children communicate through their art, their increased symbolic capacity helps them to "develop more sophisticated and abstract means to communicate and play (or create art) with others" (Wetherby & Prizant, 2000, p. 3).

Supports for communication and self-regulation that are responsive to children's or adolescent's individual needs and sensory profiles are essential to using play and the arts in therapy. These supports, together with the therapeutic relationship, encourage exploration of materials, processes, and relationships. Sensitive use of supports for autistic children can help a child to engage more fully in play and art making. Within the creative space of play and art, children can be encouraged to try new experiences and generate new ideas. Supporting or "scaffolding" (Vygotsky, 1978) children's experience to help them succeed enables greater communication and self-regulation. Russian developmental psychologist Lev Vygotsky (1978) introduced the concept of scaffolding, or supporting children's development as they integrate new experiences and new learning and understanding. Vygotsky conceptualized children's development in a holistic way (Karpov, 2005) and stressed the importance of seeing every child both in an integrated fashion and as an individual. He emphasized the importance of supporting children's learning to help them succeed. Temple Grandin (Grandin & Moore, 2016) gives an example of how her mother encouraged her to move out of her comfort zone that illustrates how such support helps to widen experience. Her mother both appreciated young Temple's enthusiasm for a construction project and enabled her emerging ability to gather additional materials for continuing the project. That meant going to a store, and communicating with others. Grandin describes this process as a "loving push" in the direction of her interests and her growth. She described her mother's support as balancing encouragement with building her capacity for independence and new learning.

Through support from the therapist, children and adolescents can be encouraged to see themselves as actively making choices. They can be helped to move from exploring the environment and materials to creating with them. And as Rubin (2005) has suggested, "the very act of creating helps the child to learn something new about himself" (p. 120). In the process of art making, children may be exposed to pleasing or integrative sensory activities, increasing the range of what is pleasurable to them. The relaxation of pressure to produce results allows the kinaesthetic experience of art making and the sensory qualities of the materials themselves to be more fully explored and enjoyed.

Engaging autistic children and adolescents with art is a means to increase flexibility, decrease perfectionism, broaden interests, and nurture strengths. Evans and Dubowski (2001) speak of a "freer and more relaxed relationship with the art making process during art therapy" (p. 10). In therapy, the therapist attunes to the child and considers the child's rhythm of working, level of comfort and energy, and their communication: both verbal and nonverbal. Evans and Dubowski (2001) describe this as "tuning in to the children's experience as naturally and comfortably as possible" (p. 75). Such "tuning in" requires particular attentiveness and skills from the therapist. The therapist may offer supports to the child. One such support is the "third hand" (Kramer, 2000).

Kramer (2000; Gerity & Annand, 2017) describes using an intuitive and skilled "third hand" in art therapy to help a child succeed in realizing their imagined creation. The emotional support and the physical third hand intervention of the therapist help to activate the healing qualities of art making. Kramer (2000) is particularly attentive to supporting "pictorial communication that eloquently and truthfully communicates experience" (p. 48). She further describes the third hand as:

> A hand that helps the creative process along without being intrusive, without distorting meaning or imposing pictorial ideas or preferences alien to the client. The third hand must be capable of conducting pictorial dialogues that complement or replace verbal exchange.
>
> (p. 48)

Using the third hand means supporting the child or adolescent with autism in developing personal imagery and creating artwork that is rich with meaning and individual gesture, color, and images. Through helping a child or adolescent to realize their creation, and not abandon their efforts, there is more for the therapist to attend to, whether the art is discussed verbally or not. Dannecker (2017) describes Kramer at work with children, literally performing an artistic rescue operation when paintings begin to be overwhelmed with running color or clay threatens to collapse. "Rescuing" the work so that it can be shared allows for the process to unfold. The efforts involved in conceptualizing and giving form to an art product is an accomplishment, and one about which the child or adolescent can then communicate with the therapist. The therapist can help them to move more fully through the process of creating art, and into richer expression and communication. The third hand helps children and adolescents with autism through moments of feeling overwhelmed or distressed and mitigates the challenges of perfectionism.

When a child found pine cones in one of my baskets of materials, he decided he would create a creature, "a wise owl." He very carefully drew out what he wanted to make, and then drew a paper beak and feet to stick on to the pine cone. I showed him how to cut these little shapes from the paper by first cutting around his drawing, so he didn't have to manipulate such a large piece of paper. He was happy to learn this new skill, but then became visibly tense while his glued pieces stuck to his fingers. Sighing, he said, "I'm frustrated" and let met help with maneuvering the overly gluey pieces. He was able to find some humor in the situation when I got a bit of glue on my fingers as well. He then washed his hands and was able to continue. This young boy's family had

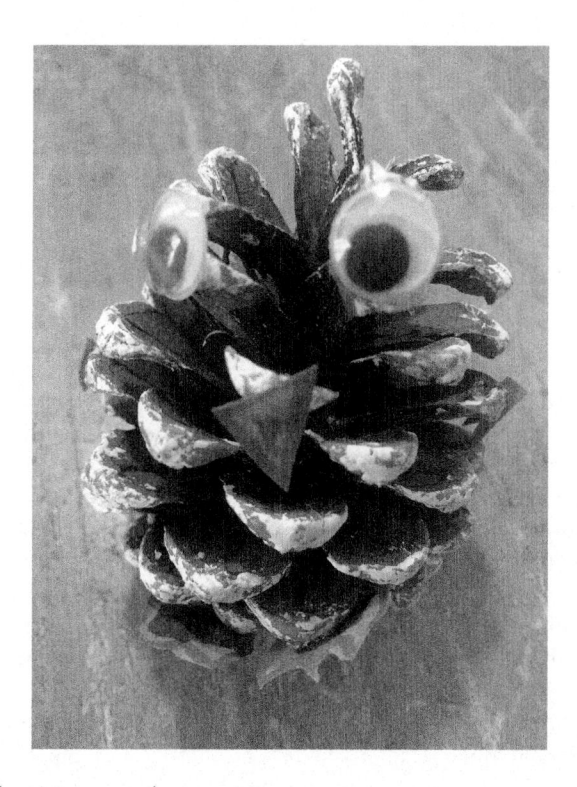

Figure 2.3 The pine cone owl.

shared that he had recent challenges with expressing anger at home. He was able to identify that frustration can feel "kind of like anger." He then realized that sharing frustration, and getting help with what is frustrating, diminishes anger. He was playful with his creation and then created a game to play with the therapist, moving the little owl around the table, exploring and looking for food and friends. He picked up an angry looking figure, and noted that he was not angry now. Without creating his own figure successfully, this perspective would not have been revealed in his play.

The "third hand" helps the creative process along without being intrusive or altering the meaning of a child's creation. The style, content, and choice of materials are the child's own. The therapist, in Kramer's view, subordinates her personal style in working with children to allow the child's own vision to take form. Seeing the work gave this child a sense of accomplishment, mastery, and satisfaction. Communication of meaning takes place both through the art and about the art, and holds possibilities for richer verbal communication as well. This child brought his art making into the realm of play, as his little owl explored the room, and he relaxed visibly as he moved with the bird.

The concept of the third hand has particularly poignant meaning for autistic children and adolescents. These children must, as Henley (2018) suggests, "be supported without being pressed too hard to maintain productivity" (p. 207). He sees art materials themselves as forming a connection with the child or adolescent (Henley, 2002). Kramer (2000) herself reflected on how,

> one of the art therapist's main occupations consists of rescuing pictures that would be destroyed for minor reasons. Again and again it has to be demonstrated that mistakes are not irreparable and that the therapist is willing and able to help at all times.
>
> (p. 49)

The third hand provides for the salvation of these drawings, paintings, and clay work, and helps children move through frustration to productivity. "Rescuing," as Kramer terms this process, is not too strong a word. I have seen children ultimately delighted with work they initially wanted to tear, crumple, or otherwise obliterate, and which did not initially seem destined to meet the child's high standards. Children need to relinquish this self-criticism to explore materials freely. I have had a child hold up a very precise drawing and ask me "How perfect is this? 75%? 95%?" This child needed to work with the challenges of perfectionism to produce work that he considered "good enough." Accepting their work and accepting the therapists' help can be a challenge for autistic children or adolescents, who, even more than other children, "may be poised between the desire to create and the fear of failure" (Kramer, 2000, p. 60).

Malchiodi's (2010) understanding of the third hand connects with what we now understand of interpersonal neurobiology (Siegel, 2012) and the growth of empathic understanding. She has observed how, "the third hand in art therapy echoes what Siegel refers to as 'mindsight,' a capacity for insight (knowing what one feels) and empathy (knowing what others feel)" (Malchiodi, 2010).

Sensitive use of the third hand encourages communication (verbal or nonverbal) as well as creation, and supports the growth of a more developed sense of self. The third hand helps children through the processes of making art and sharing art, and helps create space for therapists to attune to and listen to children.

Understanding the range of supports for an individual child can help a therapist to offer an autistic child or adolescent the "third hand" where it is needed. This support helps a child move more fully into art making, expression, and communication, and away from sensory discomfort and perfectionism. If flexibility, creativity, and meaningful communication are seen as essential therapeutic goals for children, approaches to treatment grounded in the richness of expressive languages offer a path to reaching these goals. As Greenspan and Shanker (2004) have observed, as children "become more creative, they also become more capable of making inferences and engaging in higher level abstract thinking because these also depend on generating new ideas" (p. 222). De Domenico (in Richardson, 2012) describes how "living language, living symbols" (p. 211) are created through play and art making. And Greenspan and Shanker (2004) discuss the significance of "emotionally significant charged expressive language" (p. 213) that helps a child to connect "their own emotions . . . to their symbols." Such an affective connection motivates children to use language to communicate and deepen their relationships and understanding. When a child is actively playing or creating, their sense of self-efficacy and self-awareness is supported by the presence of the therapist. Through play and art, therapists can experience children's worlds together with them.

As Schadler and De Domenico (2012) have described, when entering the play "world" that has been created, therapists must move "gently into language to develop a story after it is experienced on a deep level," (p. 90) scaffolding the ability and the willingness to communicate. Badenoch (2008) further describes the unfolding of the process taking place in play therapy, wherein "both people listen . . . with their whole bodies . . . as the symbolic world unfolds into words" (p. 220). For children and adolescents with autism, this deep listening allows therapists to attune to what they may not always hear.

Chapter 3

A Strong Image of the Child With Autism

Sitting at my art table placed between two tall windows, and choosing colors to draw with, a young child looked up from his paper and asked me, "why is art special?" In order to meet any child where she or he is, and to connect with the child through shared creative activity, that activity must be engaging and "special" to the child. The therapy setting itself must feel safe to them. When a child is actively creating or playing, the sense of self-efficacy and self-awareness the child experiences is encouraged by the presence of the therapist. The careful attention of the therapist, the acknowledgment of the process of creation, and the creation itself support relationship and communication.

Therapists need to be attuned to all the gestures, expressions, and creations that children may share. The educators of Reggio Emilia, Italy, understand that for children, there are at least "100 Languages" (Reggio Children, 1987) through which children explore their experience and understanding of the world. All children have the potential to explore their world, and to invent imaginative worlds. The expressive languages children use to discover and "invent" their worlds are a rich resource for therapists. Helping children to find their own "language," whether visual, musical, or poetic, is an important challenge. It may be difficult to know what an individual child will respond to, or in what way she or he will choose to communicate. In Reggio, the use of the word "languages" is used to capture "the fluid processes of interpersonal communication" (Goebl-Parker & Richardson, 2011, p. 74) and the capacities of the environment to support children's relationships and ideas. Therapists, suggests Orbach (2020), also must "speak many metaphorical languages . . . and synthesize them to have a fuller and richer palette of information regarding their clients" (p. 12).

When I travelled to Reggio Emilia for an International Study Group in 2008, I had studied and worked with this concept of languages for many years, first at my child's school, and later, applying these ideas about materials and languages in my therapy practice. While I was the only art or play therapist present at this global event, I nevertheless felt as if I were speaking a common language with my colleagues. This way of seeing the potential of children and the significance of children's expression resonated deeply with the way that I worked as a therapist. As I saw the documentation of "children with special rights," as children with special needs are referred to in Reggio, I better understood this resonance. The educators presented a film of a preschooler with autism. Fascinated by fish, he patiently created a school of transparent fish and slid them gently into the water in a sink in his classroom. A little girl came closer to observe, and quietly went to get a rubber fish to "swim" amongst his school. The two children played together, drawn closer through sharing of creation and play (Goebl-Parker & Richardson, 2011, p. 78). As Winnicott (2005) describes, "in playing . . . the individual child or adult is able to be creative" (p. 54). Therapists, like teachers, can connect with this unfolding creative process through using children's preferred languages.

For many children, including children with autism, as Soncini (in Gandini & Kaminsky, 2005) explains, children's difficulty with creative expression through spoken language must be supported by other opportunities to communicate. When given an opportunity to express their intentions and ideas through materials and art making, through movement, music, or play, all children can show up within the group of their peers and build relationships with them.

A strong image of the child, explains Rinaldi, (in Goebl-Parker & Richardson, 2011) supposes the concept of the child as an individual filled with "capacity, competency, and ideas" (p. 79). The philosophy and the way of Reggio Emilia is to respect the potential of each child, embracing his or her own "special" differences, qualities, and interests. When the Reggio preschools became the first in Italy to fully include children with disabilities and their families, their differences were embraced as a way of understanding these children more fully and making them an integral part of the community. In Reggio, the focus has not been on what children cannot do, but on what they could do, given supportive relationships and appropriate environments. The phrase "children with special rights" is used in Reggio to connote an image of children, including autistic children, as being capable and having potential. This image of the child is both active and interactive, as teachers or therapists look carefully at the children with whom they work to better understand each child's potential. Children's rights and strengths, rather than their needs, are examined first; and in this context support for all children is a given. In Reggio, knowledge of the child with special rights goes beyond their diagnosis or challenges to include interaction between the school, the family, and the health care system to offer holistic support. The Reggio educators feel that to focus first on children's needs risks limiting our idea of the child's potential and the ways in which they can become a member of the group.

Among the rights of all children is the right to experience the aesthetic dimension of life and the expanded possibilities offered by engaging with the languages of art, music, and movement. Art and creativity are seen as present in daily life. The concept of a "right to experience beauty" (Vecchi, 2010, p. 82) provides an environment for children in which they can feel cared for and which is supportive of psychological well-being and growth. For children with autism, this potential for movement between different languages is very significant. Different materials allow for different representations of their ideas, interests, and understanding. New materials and experiences can give children the ability to transform their environment and search for their own most natural forms of expression.

Every child has an individual profile of interests, preferences, and strengths as well as challenges. These differences may suggest new ways of supporting children and helping to build relationships. With children whose strengths are not verbal, educators are moved to look at other ways children may have of communicating. While always acknowledging individual needs for structure and support, the Reggio approach to including children involves building on the strengths of each child. A Reggio classroom offers opportunities for exploration through movement, in a setting rich in visual stimuli and offering a variety of materials for communication. Children encounter a wide range of possibilities. They are presented with many opportunities to express their ideas and share their emotional responses to life in the classroom. Teachers (like therapists) must observe these contexts and expressions carefully. With children who may not speak, who do not communicate their wants with words, Rinaldi (2007) suggests that "I (as the teacher) just have to open my eyes" to the differences between the adult's point of view and that of the child.

Engaging children in a group allows them to show up in the group in their own individual way, and allows for greater reciprocity with other children. When I worked as consultant to an early childhood program, the teachers and I observed carefully to find the preferred activities and games of a three-year-old boy with autism. We made a picture book of his favorite games, which included his favorite of rolling a ball down a slide, to be caught by a teacher or friend. Children wanted to play the games they saw in the book, and of course, the "inventor" of the game was always an important part of this process.

When visiting an older child in school for an art therapy session, I experimented in one session with teaching her a new "visual language," that of creating simple pop-ups with paper and scissors, as she told a story about dinosaurs, one of her special interests. Adeptly, she took her own scissors and began creating a tiny book to tell her story of friendship with a little dinosaur. This interest was not necessarily shared by her peers, who had mostly moved beyond the dinosaur fascination stage. Yet when she returned to the classroom, the children sitting around her were delighted by her new creation, and wanted to learn how to make a pop up as well. With my encouragement, and that of the teacher, she was able to show the others what she had done, and gather together two other children to work with her. New materials, however simple, can offer a concrete way to transform and represent the child's thoughts and reality, and to share them with others. This child had moved from exploring friendship with a mythical creature to sharing it with her peers. There is a sense of belonging that comes as a group creates together—a sense of true inclusion that is built as other children use their ability to connect with, and understand the meaning and intention expressed by the child with special rights. For the second grader I worked with, her particular strength in visual expression gave her a way to connect with others in a new way. It is validating for children to look at what they have made in the context of relationship, and to deepen relationships through sharing their creations and stories. At the end of our time together, this little girl made me an intricate paper bracelet. She told me, "everyone will know this is from someone who really likes you."

Play creates community, although reciprocal play with others can be a challenge for children on the autism spectrum. Children's play scenarios and art creations invite us to experience their world together with them, especially when we are mindful of seeing what we may not hear and remain attuned to their stories. Such personal narratives, as Siegel (Siegel & Hartzell, 2013) explains, tell stories in such a way that they help children to make sense of both their internal and external worlds, regardless of how young they may be.

Therapists working with the languages of art and play are in a unique position to engage the mind, brain, and senses, and to support children in telling their stories. Play can lead into making art. Play, as Malchiodi and Crenshaw (2017) explain, precedes creative expression through art: "Developmentally, play exists before formal artistic expression; in the earliest months of life, infants learn play through rhythm and tempo, social interactions with others through body language and sounds . . . and other sensory-based relationships with caregivers" (p. 9). Through experience, children develop the ability for imaginative, dramatic play, and also the cognitive and motor skills needed for art making. And for some children, sharing interests or artistic creations helps lead to reciprocal play. Whether through creating or playing, engagement with others generates fuller inclusion through shared experience, allowing children to enter more fully into, and contribute to, the culture of their classroom. The success of the community hinges on the recognition of the intelligence and creativity of all children as members of that community. While, as Rinaldi (in Gandini & Kaminsky, 2005) has explained, there are many ways of looking at children, many of these focus on the child's needs rather than on their strengths. Identifying children's interests, strengths, and inclinations is an essential component of altering this image to create a strong image of the child and value the contributions of all children.

Whether as teachers or as therapists, adults need to listen carefully to children. The schools of Reggio Emilia value a way of being with children that supports communication with children through a wide variety of expressive languages. Careful listening to children enables a responsive and creative way of interacting with them. These are therapeutic values as much as they are essential to learning. In the schools of Reggio Emilia, therapeutic work is integrated into the life of the school. But therapists who work with children in other settings can also embrace the idea of languages and the careful observation that is integral to the work of Reggio educators.

On a classroom observation visit one day, a young boy I worked with spontaneously asked me to be a part of his class sharing circle. He sat me down, and then announced, "guys, this is Dr. Jane. She helps me with my feelings when I get mad." After this exchange, I became very popular with the class. My client was appreciated by his peers for sharing a situation that was challenging for many of the children. I found a book about feelings in the bookcase and read it aloud to a small group of children, including the boy I had come to see.

Kaplan (2016) has discussed the importance of balancing the internal process of change through therapy with the social action goal of outer change in the environment and within relationships. "After all," as Kaplan (2018) explains further, "art therapy endeavors to facilitate internal, individual change, and social action strives to make outer, collective, difference." This relational shift in their learning and social environment is crucial for children and adolescents with autism.

Therapists can embrace a way of being with and working with children that goes beyond approaches or techniques, supporting children in a fuller expression of self and a renewed ability to communicate and connect with others. Crenshaw (2011) suggests that therapy with children gains from a frame of reference broad enough to take into account both the individual lived experience of the child and the broader context of their lives in their families, schools, and communities. He further suggests that, "an important part of making a safe place where the child can explore and eventually tell their own story is the therapist's way of being with the child." In therapy, the language of feelings plays a central role in the telling of stories that heal. The therapist's invitation to children to engage with expressive materials is also an invitation to help children access the language to convey emotions. Whether as teachers or as therapists, adults need to listen carefully to children. As Junge (2007) has explained, "the issue of *language* is an important one to all therapists," and spoken language is often "what is valued and desired" and yet the individual expression of creativity and understanding "can come in many colors, and not in words at all" (p. 45).

Therapy helps a child to find their own voice, whether this voice is heard through words or not. Art, play, movement, and music are languages for therapy as they are for learning.

Providing children and adolescents with an environment and materials that support rich expression is particularly significant for children or adolescents with autism. While the finished artwork, the product, may reflect their special and dearly held interests, and be an important focus for communication, the sensory nature of the process of creating can be soothing, engaging, or stimulating, and offer opportunities for interaction with the therapist and with others. Kaplan (2007) has discussed the essential process of balancing inner change created through therapy with the social action goal of achieving outer change (p. 11). She explains that, "we cannot separate the people we treat from the cultural settings in which they live" (p. 16). Therapy must connect with the larger world of the child, enlivening and expanding their experience. As children or adolescents gain greater flexibility and more communication skills through therapy, their wish to connect with others, and to play and share with them, can be expressed in the context of their schools and community. Listening to all children and adolescents, and allowing them the opportunity to show, as well as say, what they want and how they feel, allows them to be helpers and friends as well as learners and to experience themselves in a new way that enriches everyone's experience.

Sharing interests and experiences unifies the individual and the social realms. For children and adolescents with autism, the therapeutic environment can help to create comfort within which to explore and connect with others. Vygotsky (1978), whose sociocultural theory of child development informs the work of Reggio Emilia educators, introduced the essential developmental concept of scaffolding, or supporting children's growth as they integrate new experiences and new learning and understanding. He understood the creative nature of how the imagination unfolds within the context of the environment and relationship, and how children share their creations and imaginings with others. Vygotsky (in Penfold, 2019) as Penfold explains acknowledges how, ". . . the more a child sees, hears, and experiences, the more he knows and assimilates, the more elements of reality he will have in his experience, and the more productive will be the operation of his imagination" (p. 1).

Scaffolding children's experience by offering supports for communication and self- regulation tailored to individual children's specific needs and sensory profiles is essential for children and adolescents with autism. Individualized supports give all children freer access to multiple languages for expression and encourage communication. Sensitive, individualized use of supports for autistic children can help the child to enter more deeply into play, art making, expression, and communication. Within the creative space of play and art, children can try new experiences and generate new ideas.

The zone of proximal development as conceptualized by Vygotsky (1978) illuminates the processes whereby children are able to move beyond what they already know to develop new ideas and abilities that are developmentally ready to emerge, but not yet present. He believed that play "contains all developmental tendencies in a condensed form and is itself a major source of development" (p. 102). For a child with autism, in the context of therapy, as Dolphin observed, these abilities might include, "new interpersonal skills, an increased capacity to play or a move towards symbolic expression" (p. 143).

Scaffolding and transactional support are important elements of therapy with autistic children, even as they are essential elements of supporting their play, communication, and learning. Sensitive use of supports for autistic children can help children to organize and orient themselves. Understanding supports for the autistic child helps the therapist in offering a child a supportive "third hand" (Kramer, 2000; Gerity & Annand, 2017) where needed, to help the child move more fully into expression and communication, and away from sensory discomfort and perfectionism. Wetherby et al. (2000) suggest that, "clinicians and educators must expand their role . . . to supporting others in growth-inducing interactions and activities designed to enhance children's developmental capacities" (p. 213). When children on the autism spectrum embrace play, there can be a parallel growth in creative expression. Wolfberg (2003) developed structured "integrated play groups" to help children on the autism spectrum develop the ability for shared play. Her integrated playgroups model is in part inspired by Vygotsky's view of play as instrumental for symbolic representation and understanding the social world. In this view, play is an integral part of how children both construct knowledge and enter into their culture. However, autistic children's play style often tends to lead to their isolation from the culture of their peers, and may not encourage shared meaningful activity. Because their play may be repetitive, and involved with elaborate routines or the pursuit of narrow interests, there can be a lack of both spontaneous play with peers and the overtures that lead to reciprocal play. On the other hand, entering into play initiated by another child is also a challenge, as children with autism may not initially understand the other child's intention or interest. Thus, for children with autism, "constructing shared meaning" (Wolfberg, 2003, p. 28) through the process of play must be nurtured.

As Wolfberg (2003) observes, there is evidence to suggest that children with autism are not simply devoid of any desire to interact with peers, but rather that they lack experience with the social skills necessary to connect through shared play. The playgroup is a place where children's play skills can grow while they are supported, or scaffolded, in Vygotsky's term, by the presence of an adult. Scaffolding within the playgroup involves the provision of adjustable and temporary support structures which help support the child in using and developing new knowledge and understanding. Initially, children need more help to enter into shared play, but gradually children are able to play more freely on their own. Wolfberg has suggested the particular importance of careful observation of the expressive play of children on the autism spectrum, paying especially close attention to the symbolic dimension of play. Play and art making, coupled with a sense of safety and comfort, can lead children to richer expression and communication, what Wolfberg poetically terms, "Budding flowers of imagination . . . conveying meaning through verbal and visual images in stories and pictures" (p. 134).

Through careful observation of children's communication, both verbal and nonverbal, adults can remain flexible and responsive, modifying their own behavior in response to children's needs. Therapists can structure their environment to support children, much in the way of Reggio educators who think of the environment as a "third teacher," containing many possibilities for expression and growth.

Chapter 4

Finding a Language for Feeling

A young boy drew a smiling face in the damp sand, and then we walked together around the room and identified smiling figures in my sandtray collection.

He wanted me to help him find who was smiling and who was not. He then chose the frowning or "mad" looking figures, with some amusement, and started to play out the interaction between the smiling and frowning characters he had chosen in the sand. As Prizant (2015) has observed, while emotions are experienced, and "if anything . . . magnified" by children with autism, "their challenge is understanding and expressing their own emotions and reading the emotion in others" (p. 124). Thus a therapeutic goal for children and adolescents with autism, which Henley (2018) describes as a "core cognitive intervention" (p. 55) is to help them to "restate that which has just occurred— whether it be narrating back the content of a picture, or, in a social context, processing what they feel just occurred" (ibid). This child was able to make connections to his own life, and to the things that made him happy or left him feeling angry. He ended his play with drawing a smiling character on paper, as he had in the sand. He left the room relaxed and smiling.

Some children will not initially respond to art materials. Instead, they may readily communicate through using instruments, puppets, or the sand tray and expressive figures. A delightful preschooler and his mother listened carefully to one another as we played drums together. We moved through the space with colorful silk scarves, and created piles in which he could hide. His mother and I could find him and he could find us. While art materials were always present, and sometimes gently offered, they were not the way for us to work together at this time. We connected with one another through the playful and interactive use of music and movement.

After exploring materials together, children often turn to making art, as a tangible record of this time together, and of their ideas and intentions. When combined with a flexible and playful approach, art making becomes animated, allowing for movement, change, elaboration, and exchange. Stories, rhythms, play, and building "worlds" in the sand tray, or around the room, are all ways to explore a child's story and feelings. When children do not have language available to them to express their feelings, or to describe their sensations, as

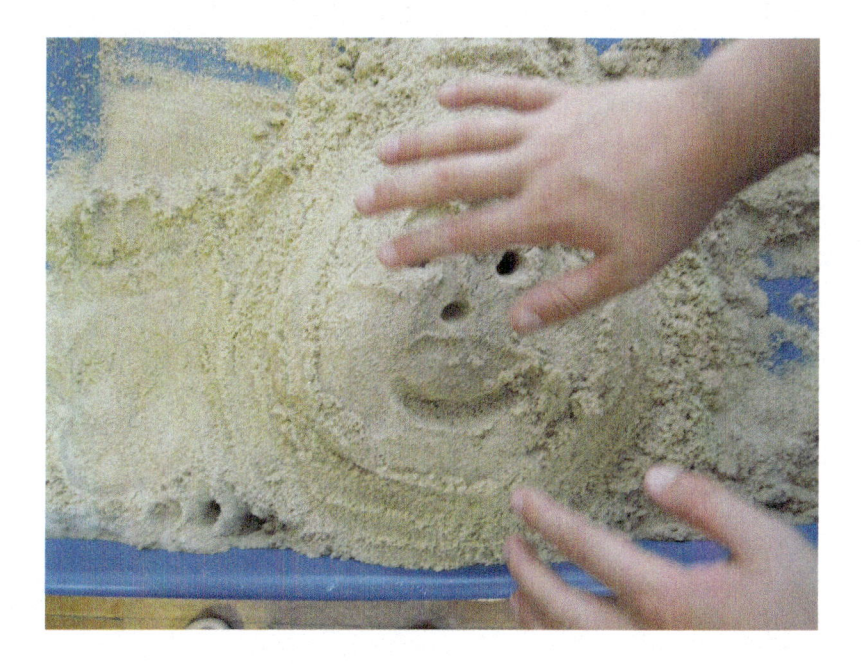

Figure 4.1 A child smooths the wet sand to draw a smiling face.

Malchiodi (2020) has explained, the inability to articulate how they are feeling and what they are experiencing can be dysregulating. Expressive "languages," then, are critically important.

Children rely on information from their senses to understand their experience and process their feelings. Grandin (2013) has explained that "our five senses are how each of us understands everything that isn't us" (location 953). And Malchiodi (2020) describes how the elements of expressive arts approaches actively draw on the senses to support expression, understanding, and communication. She explains how the sensory and movement-based elements "of rhythm, movement, enactment, visual imagery, touch and sound found in expressive arts naturally involve active participation . . . and can enhance self-regulation" (p. 168).

In therapy, the interests and emotions of a child with autism may first appear in the sand, a material that can help children to self-regulate even while it supports expression. Sometimes the sand and the figures for play provide the medium through which a verbal story emerges (Richardson, 2012) and takes on a deeper affective dimension. And sometimes play in the sand leads to further expression through drawing, painting, or clay.

For one nine-year-old boy, the sand tray was the initial space for exploring the looming challenges of the new school year. He created a literal "bridge" from the present year to the next in the sand (Richardson, 2012). We then explored ways of crossing this bridge successfully. He embodied the supports he would need through his play in the sand. We talked about his expectations of the new class and the new teacher, and we worked on ways of calming his fears of what would change. He shared the ideas he had generated through his play, and through our work together, with his parents. Then, in the following session, he carefully crafted a smiling Statue of Liberty from clay, painting her meticulously down to the shine of her torch. She stood, he said, "for new things," waiting to be experienced. As we looked together at his creation he talked about why he liked her so much, and why she was so important to him. He decided that the Statue of Liberty gave people an opportunity "to do new things" in a new country. "It's fun," he said, to play in the sand and work with clay. "I like it. It gives me the freedom to do new things." The freedom of the sand tray had helped him to find more freedom and flexibility within himself during a time of transition that originally felt overwhelming. These new feelings made him think about the experiences lying ahead that he could look forward to, and he felt more ready to enjoy them.

While another nine-year-old was always happy to come and play, he did not choose to draw, paint, or work with clay. He did not gravitate to the sand tray to tell a story. These materials were not inherently appealing to him. While a goal for him was to deepen expressive communication, he was not always responsive to the materials and media traditionally used in art or play therapy to explore thoughts and feelings. He preferred music and movement. His choice for the sand tray was to enjoy the sand's sensory properties on his speedy transit to another part of the room, and to another activity. Over time, he connected with me, learned coping skills, and became increasingly engaged with his environment, his peers, and the supportive adults in his life. I witnessed him becoming a keen observer of his environment, sharing his observations and experiences with others, and learning to communicate his preferences and needs. In the process he moved to increasing independence at school. His play was interactive and often delighted, with a pleasure that was infectious.

He explored materials, as children with autism may do, in a highly individual way. Daniel Tammet, the well-known author and artist with autism, is perhaps describing some of this child's sensations and perceptions of the sand in his remembrance of his own preschool experience:

> And when I went to kindergarten (nursery, we would say in Britain) I would love playing with sand and taking grains of sand in the sand pit and putting them through my fingers and playing with sand timers and watching the sand flow and just experimenting with this incredibly strange, weird, but strangely beautiful thing we call reality, this world. The fact that if you take a tube and you put a ball in one side it will come out the other side. It's just an obvious thing to most people but to me growing up during early childhood it wasn't obvious that if you put a ball in one side

of a tube, it will come out the other side. All these kinds of little experiments to discover the laws of how this strange but beautiful world actually worked.

(In Kaufman, 2012)

Children's preference for musical and rhythmic activities makes sense developmentally. Grandin (1996) feels that, "musical and rhythmic activities are highly recommended for autistic children" (p. 151). Dance therapist Suzi Tortora (2006) describes how the movement of the body tells stories through "a dialogue between self and surroundings" (p. 75) that precedes verbal language.

Different expressive languages may be seen as different ways in which children are drawn to explore themselves and share their thoughts and feelings. Adults can get to know a child more fully by looking beyond materials or techniques, to examine the "processes of empathy and intense relations" (Vecchi, 2010, p. 12) made visible through the use of movement, play, or experimenting with open-ended materials. In their preferences for a particular expressive approach or language, children with autism are as varied as any children.

Young children are typically able to move from one expressive language to another, a propensity that is to be encouraged for autistic children as this supports them in gaining greater flexibility. The growth of expression, "finds sources from play, as well as from practice . . . in fact, drawing, painting (and the use of all languages) are experiences and explorations of life, of the senses, and of meanings" (Gandini et al., 2005, p. 9) including emotional meanings. Children may be drawn to use a particular range of experiences and materials for expression and building connection. As music therapist Krystal Demaine has observed, "whether the modality be art, dance, music . . . the key is to speak the language of these children. I think that the arts offer sensory-motor integrative experience that can allow for social reciprocity and the exchange of language that individuals with autism speak" (personal communication, March 30, 2012). Through observing and listening carefully to children, therapists may find that access to richer visual expression and spoken language may come first through movement, music, and play. The key to working with an individual child is to be attuned to that child's creative and expressive language, as well as to the child's state. Gaskill and Perry (2014) describe how understanding both "the real developmental capabilities of the child and the child's current state" (p. 179) are the essential precursors to effectively using play in a truly therapeutic and developmentally appropriate fashion.

As communication is established through the arts and play, working with responsive and flexible materials encourages flexibility. Exploration of new materials and new experiences supports communication and expression of emotion. One seven-year-old was ready to deepen this process of exploration. His ability to observe and interact with others had given rise to a fascination with moods, especially the presence of tears, and what these tears might mean. He would trace the path of tears on his own face, or his mother's face, and search for tears in her expression, or his own as he looked into the mirror. Shore (in Ariel & Naseef, 2005) describes his own early experience with the emotions of others in a way that might offer a clue to what this child was experiencing in his fascination with tears:

> Often I find myself fusing with other people's emotions. My parents taught me that 'people are not mind reader' and that if you have a feeling you need to state it. As a result, whenever I have an emotion that seems out of context with the environment I have to look around and verbalize it to another person.
>
> (p. 202)

Shore mentions picking up on the anxiety of others and having to identify whether an emotion "is or is not coming from me" (ibid).

This child's mother and I both wondered about the source of his interest in tears, and searched for ways to help him identify his own emotions. His mother wisely showed him the difference between happy tears of pride and sad tears, letting him know that it helps to talk or ask questions about a feeling. She built on his fascination with faces and helped him to explore feelings.

In therapy, I wanted to hear his stories. I wanted to help him understand the changeable nature of feelings so that he would not feel "stuck" in sadness. I wanted to explore whether there were events in his life that were causing him sadness that he had not expressed. I wanted to help him with identifying and expressing feelings, which could also help him at the times he felt stressed at school. We both hoped to give him alternatives for greater self-regulation and to increase the appropriateness of supports when he needed them.

In our play together, he was cheerful, smiling, and responsive, as we looked at one another's faces and identified how we were feeling. Together with his mother, we looked at one another and identified the source of our smiles as happiness in having fun together. When we played a game with scarves, taking turns at covering one another, he smiled from the middle of a pile of silk. "How are you feeling?" his mother and I asked, and he replied, "happy." Here is where we began to explore the broader range and expression of affect, first through play, then through music, and later through art.

As we played the drums, we asked "who is happy to hear our music?" with the child enthusiastically replying as he shared his rhythm. At this point in the therapy, he began spending more time in the office without his mother, smilingly asking her, "are you going to leave?" once he had settled into the room on each visit. He also moved into more complex play.

He thoroughly explored the materials for movement and music: balls, scarves, drums, and xylophones. We began to play together in an increasingly reciprocal fashion. Where my musical ball maze had initially been so beguiling and absorbing that I sometimes had to hide it away for the first part of a session, lest we do nothing but listen to its chiming, now we played a game that he had originated, taking turns putting the balls through the maze, where they would hit a xylophone key. While one of us made music with the maze, the other played a xylophone in harmony with the sounds the balls created as they rolled downward. His acute ear always served to let me know if I was off pitch, and he allowed me, or even a puppet, to take turns playing.

He also responded positively when I offered an invitation to play in the sand, or to draw. He began telling stories about his play in the sand, and also to talk about his drawings, happily declaring, "I'm an artist" as he settled in to draw. We worked back and forth, from art to play. His drawing and his play in the sand tray helped him develop the stories he told, and their greater connection to his own feelings. He drew a baseball player in a Red Sox hat, who was sad at a loss, but then happy at a win. He drew his own face, in tune with the emotions of his favorite team.

His play in the sand tray moved from sifting sand, without much interest in adding any images, to searching for the images he liked. He used these images to share his special interests. In creating his first sand tray with figures, he chose a Red Sox player and a bridge, two things that fascinated him. He then added a little boy who watched the scene.

He had created his first story in the sand. This simple but eloquent "world" in the sand, with the choice of a boy like him, brought this child more fully

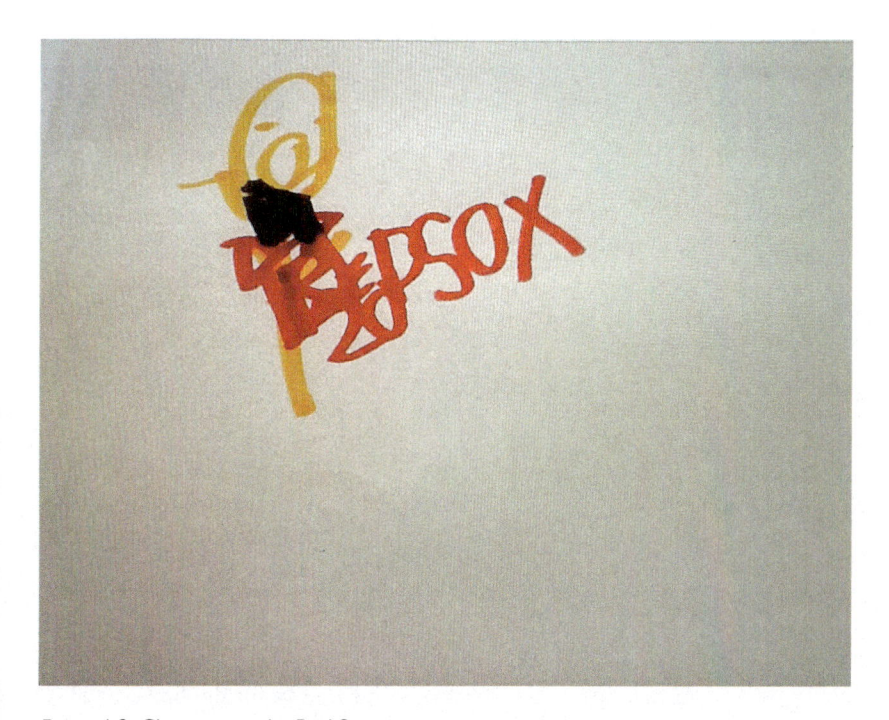

Figure 4.2 Cheering on the Red Sox.

into his story. This child did not need to tell this story in words, and indeed he did not, but the sense of drama and relationship between the figures he had chosen was clear. Later, he would share more of the experiences and intentions taking place for his characters and within their world. As we continued to play, and then to draw, his stories began to have more movement and become more complex. He was able to move outward from his intense focus.

Connecting with special interests, or fixated interests, is an important part of allowing children to feel comfortable in the therapy setting and relationship. Special interests, when met with interest from an adult, offer another window into the child's thoughts. "As a rule," as Grandin (1996) observes, "therapists object to catering to fixations. But many fixations in autistic type children have to do with a need for reducing arousal in an over-active nervous system" (p. 113). When children feel more regulated, they are increasingly able to engage with others.

One day, this child picked up one of the Red Sox figures and declared, "he's sad . . . he hurt his leg." He placed the player in the sand tray. "Who can help him?" I asked. Together we found a doctor, and added her to the scene. A story unfolded of the player getting a shot, and then starting to feel better, even though he was "embarrassed" about getting a shot. He decided that "number

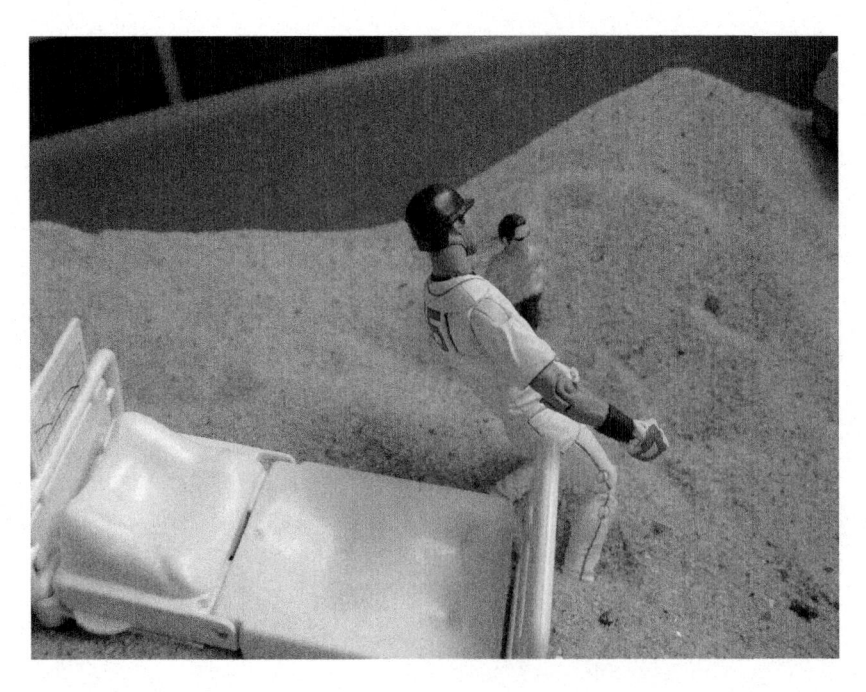

Figure 4.3 The hurt player.

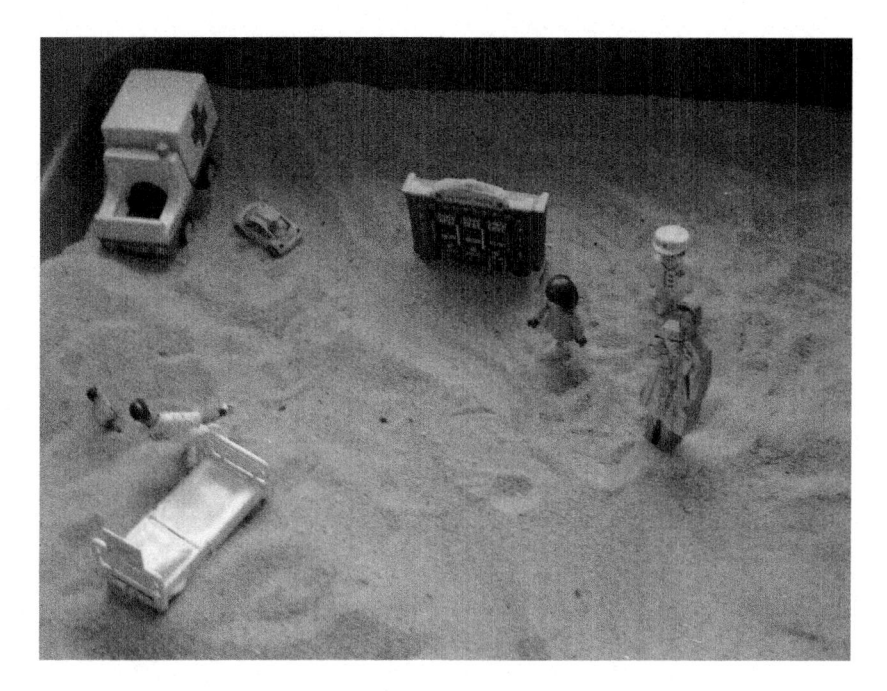

Figure 4.4 The helpers in the sand.

16, Dustin Pedroia" was now feeling better, and the play began to move more quickly and become more complex.

Fenway Park went into the sand tray, together with another favorite thing, a yellow VW bug. He had used these "punch buggies" to explore feelings before, saying, "Punchy is sad," and then mimicking the face and sinking body of sadness himself. He portrayed "sad" very effectively. But in this sand tray, he parked his favorite car beside the park, and chose a man in a yellow shirt to stand beside it. His team had won and all were feeling happy. We had been working on identifying feelings as connected to events and relationships, feelings shared with and supported by others, and working toward a greater awareness of feelings as states that can change. The sand tray was a place to explore the feelings evoked by his stories as they unfolded.

As he explored narratives in his play, his drawings became more expressive as well, and he took more pleasure in creating them. He drew his own experiences of traveling, swimming, and sharing pleasurable experiences with his family. His favorite vocabulary of images, including bridges and cars, were integrated into drawings depicting his experience of driving over a bridge on the way to an enjoyable vacation. He drew himself smiling as he rode bikes with his mother. His special interests were engaged both in his art and his play,

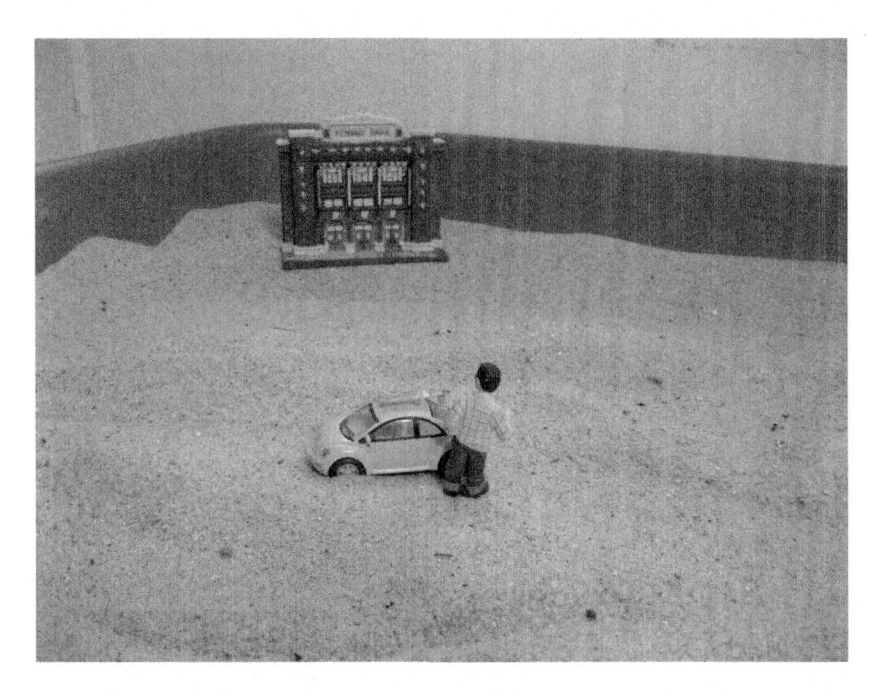

Figure 4.5 Anticipating the game, and a favorite car.

but he was able to broaden these interests, and his range for recognizing and expressing affect as he told his stories.

He used different visual and expressive languages "as a means for investigating the world and building bridges and relationships between different experiences and languages" (Giudicci in Vecchi, 2010, p. 57). When children investigate their experience in the world, making their thoughts and feelings visible through art or symbolic play, they can begin to talk about their experiences and emotions. Through valuing and supporting children's experiences and interests, adults support the development of a positive self-representation for the child. A child's painting or clay figure, their musical explorations, their dramas and their play, form a living document of the child's feelings and ideas. These are the tools for growth and change. Helping children to find their own "language," whether visual, musical, or poetic, is an important challenge. As children share their stories, whether they speak or remain silent, their world of the senses and feelings expands and becomes increasingly relational.

Chapter 5
Who Is Diagnosis For?

The ways that autism is discussed have changed along with the process and criteria for making a diagnosis of autism. The use of more fluid language, referring alternatively to autistic people and to people with autism, which is now used to more accurately describe what Mundy (2020) has called, "this individual difference that we call autism," is one significant reflection of this dynamic change. Being "on the spectrum" is a concept that has evolved since Kanner's (1943) early diagnostic description of a child exhibiting ". . . an abstraction of mind which made him perfectly oblivious to everything about him" (p. 218). The current concept of an autism "spectrum," as Grandin (2017) describes it, is vast, encompassing a range "from Einstein to a person who does not talk." Moreover, there is no firm dividing line at the ends of the "spectrum" since, as Mundy (2020) notes, the way that autism is viewed has changed over time.

Autism "is a very heterogeneous condition" (Bolte, 2020). It has been discussed as a different way of being human, but also as a disability and a disorder. Brown (2019), who writes from the perspective of an autistic advocate, describes how:

> Autism . . . is not a disease. It is a neurological, developmental condition; it is considered a disorder, and it is disabling in many and varied ways. It is lifelong . . . It is an edifying and meaningful component of a person's identity, and it defines the ways in which an individual experiences and understands the world around him or her. It is all-pervasive.
>
> (para. 11)

Chown (2019) suggests that non-autistic individuals have as much difficulty in understanding autistic minds as the reverse, and suggests that therefore the term "disability" is not used appropriately when part of the criteria being used for this categorization of autism is a lack of understanding of others. Walker (2014) further maintains that, while "autism is still widely regarded as a 'disorder,' this view has been challenged in recent years by proponents of the neurodiversity model, which holds that autism and other neurocognitive variants are simply part of the natural spectrum of human biodiversity" (p. 1).

Given the broad range of people with autism, the different conceptualizations of what autism actually is, and the reality that diagnosis is one of the most controversial aspects of clinical practice, an essential starting point for understanding autism is looking at individuals and at what is possible for them. For clinicians working with autistic people, it is critically important to focus on the specific needs and preferences of individuals whether they are adults or, as in my practice, children and adolescents. "Our goal," as Shore (2006a) explains, "should be to help persons with autism understand and use their strengths to work around any presenting challenges so they, just like everyone else, have an equal chance at living a fulfilling and productive life" (p. 203).

Attwood (2006) describes how the child or adolescent with autism, similar to many of my own clients, typically "has a clinically significant difficulty with the understanding, expression, and regulation of emotion" (p. 29) and is thus, as Kim et al. (2000) describe, at risk for anxiety and depressed mood. "Despite us knowing that depression among people on the spectrum is a common problem, in truth we know alarmingly little about depression and autism," as Veenstra-VanderWeele (in Weinstock, 2019) explains. This suggests that symptoms of depression and anxiety need to be carefully monitored when working with autistic adolescents and children.

Children have explained to me how they "don't want to worry so much," but they have also discussed their sense that autism is "part of me," and how their interests and focus help them to be better at doing the things they care about. Attwood (2006) has emphasized the importance of dealing with stressors to address the clinical challenges of anxiety and depression. And Cozolino (2010) discusses how support for emotional regulation and targeting stress "should always be an aspect of healing relationships" (p. 350) and further notes that the regulation of stress positively affects neuroplasticity. Addressing stressors is essential to therapy with children and adolescents with autism, as is an awareness of social and sensory challenges. As Herbert (2012) has explained, "autism involves the whole body" (p. 7). Walker (2014) describes how encompassing bodily experience is in autism.

> An autistic child's sensory experience of the world is more intense and chaotic than that of a non-autistic child, and the ongoing task of navigating and integrating that experience thus occupies more of the autistic child's attention and energy. This means the autistic child has less attention and energy available to focus on the subtleties of social interaction.
> (para. 5)

A holistic and individualized approach to therapy engages the mind, brain, and senses through art and play, creating comfort and freeing energy to connect with others. This concept of the flow of energy is present in the work of non-Western arts therapists (Richardson et al., 2012). From the Traditional Chinese Medicine perspective, as Kossak (2015) describes, therapists "tune in to the body to feel sensations and emotions" (p. 7). Such tuning in goes beyond the parameters of the prevailing diagnostic criteria for autism and addresses individual challenges in a holistic fashion.

Despite having shared challenges, individuals with autism are different from one another in important ways. The purpose of making a diagnosis of autism (needed as it is for both educational services and insurance reimbursements) is to more fully understand and meet individual needs. Yet it may sometimes seem, as Moat (2013) describes, that "autism is more of an umbrella term covering a range of possibilities, rather than a useful diagnosis in itself" (p. 10). The nature of this broad range is such that, according to Happe (2011) there is "widespread agreement that autism is a spectrum that varies among different individuals and even within individuals during their lifetime" (p. 1). Understanding individual development is thus an essential part of any diagnostic process.

Greenspan (1998) has explained how the biological processes of taking in and processing information from the world, and of responding to and connecting with the world, are both complex and individual. Understanding autism is made even more difficult, Jaswal and Akhtar (2018) suggest, by evidence that "some influential accounts of autism rest on a questionable assumption that many of its behavioral characteristics indicate a lack of social interest—an assumption that is flatly contradicted by the testimony of many autistic people themselves" (p. 1). To understand the lived experience of autistic people, it is necessary to understand both the individual's interaction with their environment and the impact of the environment and the behavior of others.

With brain imaging, as Grandin (2013) explains, it is possible to "see the biological connections between parts of the brain and many of the behaviors that make up the coherent diagnosis of autism" (loc 638). However, autism is still diagnosed through observing behavior. Insel has suggested that instead, it could be more helpful to look at the "development of the brain as a starting point in understanding autism," (in Deweert, 2013) and that this would lend greater specificity to understanding the complexity of autism.

Yet for clinicians, behavior remains significant. While most clinicians understand that autism affects the way the brain functions, a client's behavior might be causing them distress, or it might be impeding their learning and relationships. Social awkwardness, for example, "can happen even if a child's IQ is off the charts" as noted by Shore (2006b, p. 16). The way autistic children behave in a treatment setting can feel both very individual and also very different from the way children without autism behave. Their interests and preoccupations, as Shore (2006b) describes, often "go beyond the normal interests of a developing child" (p. 17). These interests can become strengths.

Barron Cohen (in Opar, 2019) suggests that "defining subtypes of autism—and their corresponding needs for support and accommodation" (p. 16) could bring a needed focus to individuals and their needs as well as help move toward a meaningful shift in the currently contentious discussion and definition of autism through balancing individual needs for acceptance and self-realization and for supports. Autistic behaviors are now gaining wider understanding and acceptance and autistic people are having a broader voice in advocacy for and understanding of autism. Silberman suggests that autistic people are "significantly different in ways that need to be understood and supported" (in Muzikar, 2016).

Prizant (2015) notes that "Autism Spectrum Disorder is now among the most commonly diagnosed developmental disabilities: the U.S. Centers for Disease Control estimates that it affects as many as one in fifty school-age children" (p. 3). Of children who received an autism diagnosis in 2014, according the U.S. Centers for Disease Control, while 85% presented with developmental concerns, only 42% were evaluated for these concerns by age three (p. 7). And while autism can be diagnosed by age two, most children were not diagnosed until age four. Accessing a diagnosis demands parental involvement and persistence, education, and may involve significant resources as well.

Two groups of children are still likely to be underdiagnosed, and thereby to be left without access to services at home and in school. Boys are four times as likely to be diagnosed with autism as are girls (CDC, 2018, p. 6). And children of color remain less likely to be diagnosed than white children (CDC, 2018). In 2014 the CDC found that white children are still more likely to be identified with ASD than black or Hispanic children (2018, p. 6). Closer analysis reveals that "white children are about 19 percent more likely than black children and 65 percent more likely than Hispanic children to be diagnosed with autism" (Furfaro, 2017, p. 1). This discrepancy is not fully explained by differences in socioeconomic status, according to Durkin (in Furfaro, 2017), who, together with her colleagues, analyzed the CDC data. Still, the numbers of children diagnosed with autism suggests that while "autism awareness and access to services are increasing across racial and ethnic groups . . . the prevalence among minority children still lags behind that of white children" (p. 1). Lack of access to diagnostic evaluation for a child with developmental concerns means that "we really just don't know what the true prevalence of this condition is, particularly among minority kids," as based on data from the CDC (ibid).

For girls with autism, as Riley-Hall (2012) explains, "because girls with autism may behave more passively than their male counterparts, some have gone undiagnosed until elementary school or later, with parents struggling to help their daughters on their own, long after the early intervention years have passed" (p. 37). While both teachers and clinicians may expect children with autism "to act out and resist when faced with frustration and confusion," (p. 38) girls may present as shy or reticent. These qualities may impede getting an accurate diagnosis. Boys who tend to internalize rather than acting out under stress also have had more trouble in receiving an accurate diagnosis, in my clinical experience. And in the case of girls who are more active and aggressive, adults "are often not prepared to see aggression and loss of control in girls because it flies in the face of stereotypes about boys' and girls' behavior" (p. 39).

The range of autism-related diagnoses that were present in the DSM IV (1994) are now contained within a single diagnosis of Autism Spectrum Disorder (ASD) in the DSM V (2013). This is one of the largest diagnostic changes in the updated manual. The American Psychiatric Association fact sheet on the ASD (2013) states that the previously separate diagnoses of autistic disorder, Asperger's disorder, childhood disintegrative disorder, and pervasive developmental disorder not otherwise specified, "were not consistently applied across different clinics and treatment centers" (p. 1). Lord (in Zeldovich, 2018) observed that "It was clear that the same child could get a PDD-NOS, Asperger or autism diagnosis from different people, depending on who diagnosed them" (p. 1). The intention behind the change was that the new ASD diagnosis should actually apply to those who were previously diagnosed with one of the other diagnoses; however, this is not always the case.

Mandy, whose work focuses on the conceptualization of autism, has suggested that retaining the terms autism or autism spectrum disorder, while understanding that it encompasses a wide range of individuals, "retains identity for those whose sense of self and insight into behaviors have been enhanced by receiving an autism diagnosis" (in Bousted, 2015).

While the autism diagnosis may now be consistent, if broad, as Grandin (2013) explains, on a biological and experiential level, "Autistic brains don't all see the world the same way" (loc. 1835). Even two very visual thinkers will not process or understand the world in the same way. For example, when Grandin (2013) looked at the art work of Jessica Park, she realized that while Park "clearly could think in pictures, just as I do . . . the pictures she saw in her mind weren't my kind of pictures" (loc. 1861). Park's imagery focuses on color and pattern in a way that is fundamentally different from Grandin's perception of structure and detail. As Shore (2006b) describes, "each diagnosed case of autism appears to have its own pattern, like a fingerprint," (p. 13) and this pattern would seem to extend to strengths as well as challenges.

Whatever the parameters of the diagnosis, autism remains complex. Porges (2011) has observed that autism is "represented by a heterogeneity of the behavioral and neurophysiological features" (p. 210) present for an individual. Brown (2011) describes a further concern with such a broad definition, noting how,

> Some people are afraid that non-speaking Autistics with lower levels of adaptive functioning skills will be overlooked with the more inclusive criteria, whereas others are afraid that highly verbal Autistics who often have higher levels of adaptive functioning skills will be overlooked with the more inclusive criteria.
> (Section 3)

And London discusses the treatment-related difficulties with the current autism diagnosis, noting that, "autism is so broad that it would be more appropriate to focus treatment programs on the problems and not on the diagnosis" (in Wright, 2015).

The current discussion of the challenges of the concept of "high functioning autism" would suggest the critical importance of this approach. Alvares describes how,

> The term '*high functioning* autism' is not a diagnostic term and is based on an IQ assessment, rather than a functional assessment. It was originally used to describe people without an intellectual disability, yet somehow has crept into everyday use and has come to imply that people can manage perfectly fine, and don't experience any everyday challenges.
> (University of Western Australia, 2019)

Regardless of accomplishment and intelligence, "high functioning" people on the autism spectrum can and do experience sensory and practical challenges on a daily basis. According to a recent study of more than 2,000 people on the spectrum (Chawla, 2019), struggles with daily living skills are prevalent among "high functioning" autistic people. Andrew Whitehouse (in Chawla, 2019), the lead investigator of this study, has noted how using the term high functioning autism disregards entirely both these struggles and the need for supports. For children, concludes Lord (2020), the levels of severity specified in the DSMV pose a potential pitfall. I have met children similar to those she describes, who are very bright, and possessed of unusual abilities in an area of interest, but who are also experiencing significant challenges. These children may have difficulty receiving an accurate diagnosis. As Lord (2020) elaborates in her consideration of outcomes for a particular child, "we've concentrated on how smart he is . . . now let's concentrate on how to make his life better."

One instrument for a more individualized and comprehensive diagnosis is the World Health Organization's ongoing project, the International Classification of Functioning (ICF, 2017), which is seen as "a tool to describe the lived experience of a person with ASD in a comprehensive and standardized way." This diagnostic tool is informed by the awareness that, as Bolte (2020) describes it, "autism is a very heterogeneous condition" with a continuum of strengths and difficulties present for individuals. Within such a balanced view of autism, there is a focus on individual experience and interaction with the environment. The WHO has stated that, "interventions for people with ASD need to be accompanied by broader actions for making physical, social and attitudinal environments more accessible, inclusive, and supportive" (WHO, 2021). Such a balanced and person-centered view of autism has not always prevailed.

A Brief History of Diagnosing Autism

Kanner's (1943) description of autism discussed the communication and relationship challenges of autism for the first time, and his definition of autism applied to a very narrow group of individuals (all of whom were children). Kanner (1943) described children who needed sameness and solitude; children who "disregarded . . . people, and instantly went for objects, preferably those that could be spun" (p. 220). He suggested emotional causes for the symptoms of autism. Kanner, explains Zeldovich (2018)

> viewed autism as a profound emotional disturbance that does not affect cognition. In keeping with his perspective, the second edition of the DSM, the DSM-II, published in 1952, defined autism as a psychiatric condition—a form of childhood schizophrenia marked by a detachment from reality.
>
> (p. 1)

His description of the children he studied discussed the communication and relationship challenges of autism for the first time. However, these challenges were seen as psychologically based, and the parents of children with autism were characterized as cold and disconnected from their children. While understanding children's relationships is essential in the diagnostic process, this understanding is very different from attributing a condition to the dynamics of a relationship when it is in fact neurologically based. Kanner's diagnostic criteria prevailed until, as Silberman (2015) describes it, Rimland's research in 1964 "consigned the theory of toxic parenting to the dustbin of history" (p. 261).

Rimland (2015) suggested the challenges of developing relationships in autism has a cognitive component. He discussed how the thought process in autism, which inhibits the ability to generalize, impacts relationships. Yet when we consider the nature of this thought process, suggests Barron Cohen (in Rimland, 2015), "what we see is not evidence of dysfunction, but rather evidence of difference" (p. 1). And Herbert's (2012) neuroanatomical study of school-age children with autism did not find "broken brain regions" in these children. Rather, she found that the brain regions are not efficiently connected. Such underconnectivity impacts communication and emotional regulation, and makes flexibility in behavior challenging. Overconnectivity between sensory areas of the brain has been observed. Toddlers with autism were found to have greater connectivity between the networks governing vision and integrating movement and sensory information (Askham, 2020). Such differences may impact overall development when, as Fishman (in Askham, 2020) describes, "Their brain is busy with things it shouldn't be busy with" (p. 1).

In moving his focus away from the intrapsychic processes in autism, Rimland searched for biological origins of autism, both genetic and environmental

(Richardson, 2016). He discussed how an understanding of the sensory system and sensory sensitivities common in autism is also critical in providing effective support for people with autism. Appropriate supports allow self-regulation, communication, and relationships to flourish.

In 1980, the DSM-III (American Psychiatric Association) described autism as a pervasive developmental disorder. Children with autism move through developmental stages, as do all children. Both Greenspan (2009) and Prizant (2015) have noted how this process is different, as well as individual, for children on the spectrum; and Prizant suggests that we can most appropriately see autism as "a different way of being human" (p. 4). These differences were initially pathologized. Kanner (1943) raised questions about the parents of the children in his sample, stating that "there were very few really warmhearted fathers and mothers" (p. 250) among them, and he considered these dysfunctional relationships a central challenge in working with children who have autism.

Rimland's (2015) later research suggested that difficulty in developing relationships has a cognitive component. He discussed how the thought process in autism impacts relationships. Autistic people, he suggested, have challenges in understanding "the concept of similarity between one's self and the model," (p. 109) which is a fundamental requirement for imitating and connecting with others and for building reciprocal relationships. His discussion of a cognitive theory remains consistent with more recent research on cognition in autism. Rimland's work (2015) thus successfully challenged an affective formulation of the diagnosis and the etiology of autism. He considered the neurobiology of autism and the role of the sensory system in autism. He believed that an understanding of the sensory system and the sensory sensitivities that are common in autism, was also critical in providing effective support for people with autism (2015) and has discussed how such "process-based," (p. 153) relational, multisensory interventions support regulation and connection for individuals with autism.

Bauman (2015) feels that Rimland's research, "laid the groundwork for the clinical work . . . which is at the forefront of our more modern approaches to the understanding of autism today" (p. 14). Herbert (2012) describes how current research related to brain connectivity and coherence is preceded by Rimland's work. Herbert (2012) further explains how in autism, "there are differences both in network connections (structural and functional connectivity) and in network hubs (particular regions of the brain with relative specializations in different functions)," (p. 274) including language, emotion processing, sensory processing, motor function, and coordination. On the basis of Rimland's work, Kanner later revised his own formulation of autism as psychological in nature, both contributing a foreword to Rimland's original research and recognizing the significance of a biologically based approach.

The current diagnosis of Autism Spectrum Disorder is made based on observation. Regardless of the instrument used, the focus is on identifying communication challenges and challenges in relating to others, and also on the presence of restricted, repetitive behaviors or interests that impact behavior. An alternative perspective on autism, explains Walker (2014), writing from the perspective of an autistic academic, is that autism "Produces distinctive, atypical ways of thinking, moving, interaction and sensory and cognitive processing. One analogy that has often been made is that autistic individuals have a different neurological 'operating system' than non-autistic individuals" (p. 1).

Capturing the strengths, challenges, and experiences of individuals, and understanding their priorities is essential to therapy with children and adolescents with autism, who, no less than adults, deserve relationships and therapeutic supports that will make a difference that is meaningful to them. Identifying what would make a personally meaningful difference for autistic people is essential in supporting their wellbeing.

For the clinician practicing with people with autism it may sometimes seem, as Moat (2013) states, that "autism is more of an umbrella term covering a range of possibilities, rather than a useful diagnosis in itself" (p. 10). In an editorial in *Trends in Neuroscience* Eric London suggests that the broadness of the current autism diagnosis makes it most helpful to focus treatment on presenting concerns. London explains how too broad a focus can impede clinical progress:

> Saying that 'social deficits' is the symptom is a problem. We're actually including many different symptoms under this same big umbrella. For example, we have social anxiety, we have lack of social cognition, we have a lack of social interest—all of these may have different origins, but they all lead to the same endpoint.
>
> (Wright, 2015)

And as Levine and Chedd (2007) note, while particular interventions may work well for certain challenges or for certain individuals at a given moment, there exists a broad range of interventions and supports that may be effective over time. These might include supports at school or work, speech therapy, occupational therapy, and psychotherapy. Walker (2014) cautions that, in psychotherapy, when therapists "have an autistic client suffering from anxiety and depression . . . remember that your job is to treat the client for anxiety and depression, not for autism."

Prizant (2015) explains that, "Autism is called a spectrum disorder because the abilities and challenges of people with autism fall along a continuum, and no two people manifest autism in the same way" (p. 223). Wing (1997) initially conceptualized the autism diagnosis as a continuum, making it, as Silberman (2015) explains, "not a categorical diagnosis but a dimensional one" (p. 351). The later concept of a spectrum evolved from this concept of an autistic continuum. When Wing and Gould observed children for autistic behaviors in 1964, notes Silberman (2015), "they couldn't help but notice a much larger group of children" (p. 349) who had similar traits to those described by Kanner, but who did not merit an autism diagnosis. These children, they found, were in some ways similar to the children described by Asperger in 1944 (Silberman, 2015). Their strengths and challenges were characterized by a diagnosis of Asperger's Syndrome as distinct from an autism diagnosis. Historically, Asperger assessed that those children who presented at the "favorable" (p. 12) end of the range of an autism diagnosis, and thus were labelled as having Asperger's Syndrome, were the children who could be educated to join more fully in society, which was his therapeutic goal for them. Asperger's broader range for conceptualizing autism, however, came with dangerous implications for those children lacking the communication skills that enabled them to attend mainstream schools.

Asperger's work was originally seen as appreciating neurodiversity, and acknowledging children's differences, according to Sheffer (2019). However, the context for Asperger's work was that of Nazi psychiatry, as practiced in the Vienna of the 1940s. The outcome for the children falling at the other end of the spectrum was dire: separation from their families, and death. Sheffer (2019), in her discussion of the tragic history of these children, warns of how "diagnoses can be shaped by social and political forces, how difficult those may be to perceive, and how hard they may be to combat" (p. 15).

When autism initially began to be seen as less rare and devastating, in part following the conceptualization of the Asperger's Syndrome diagnosis, "tens of thousands of children, teenagers, and adults . . . gained access to the educational placements and social services they deserved, for the first time in history" (Silberman, 2015, p. 41). A diagnosis of Asperger's Syndrome Pervasive Developmental Disorder NOS enabled both appropriate education and needed supports for children. However, Wing (2005), who more broadly publicized the Asperger's diagnosis in 1981 (Sheffer, 2019, p. 13), titled an article in which she discussed the heterogeneous nature of autism, "Reflections on Opening Pandora's Box." Once the more differentiated diagnostic criteria for autism spectrum disorders again disappeared, she suggested, many children who might in the past have received an Asperger's diagnosis, with attendant supports at home and at school, would now find themselves without needed services.

Children are now being diagnosed with autism at younger and younger ages, although "caution is advised in making the diagnosis in children younger than 18 months" (Zero to Three, 2016, p. 17). The DC:0–5, which is the manual for Diagnostic Classification of Mental Health and Developmental Disorders of Infancy and Early Childhood (Zero to Three, 2016) suggests that clinicians should assess children for the purpose of understanding and meeting their needs. "Any intervention," the authors suggest, "should be based on as complete an understanding of the infant/young child and the infant's/young child's relationships as it is possible to achieve" (p. 7). They also cite the importance of looking at individual strengths as well as challenges.

The *DC: 0–5* notes that, for the youngest children, "there is wide individual variation in developmental trajectories of infants/young children who develop ASD" (p. 18). The Interdisciplinary Council on Developmental and Learning Disorders (2000) suggests that in assessing children's needs it is essential to "go beyond syndrome-based approaches and build on emerging knowledge of different functional developmental patterns within broad syndromes, such as autism" (p. 4). These patterns can be identified, and understanding them helps to identify strengths and support needs.

My own experience of working in early intervention, where interdisciplinary team evaluation is the norm, first showed me the value of individualized and integrative evaluation and intervention for children, including therapy, as a part of a comprehensive program. Individualized evaluation, as Greenspan and Wieder suggest (in ICDL, 2000) moves beyond "standardized, one-time assessments to observing functional impairments in the context of truly helpful interventions over time" (p. 63). Children sharing the same diagnosis, as the ICDL Clinical Practice Guidelines note, "have very different functional developmental capacities" (p. 11) and different needs.

Bromfield (2010) discusses how, for children and adolescents, creative approaches enable movement in therapy. And Moat (2013) has found that creative approaches to therapy enable, "better emotional and communicative expression" (p. 27) for people with autism, regardless of age. Interestingly, Rimland's (Miller et al., 2015) clinical focus on autism evolved to consider the strengths and skills of people with autism. This research was informed by his experience as the parent of a child with autism, Mark Rimland, who has become an accomplished artist. Working with his visual strengths enabled his "blossoming social skills and his widening awareness of others" (Landolf, 2015) as his sister describes. Prizant (2015) suggests that such focused interests held by many on the autism spectrum, "though they come with challenges . . . often represent the greatest potential for people with autism" (p. 70). Herbert (2012) has also discussed how individuals with autism have, "hidden gifts . . . even if they are blocked by lots of confusion and difficulties," and that "people with autism are capable of creativity and insight" (p. 245). For the therapist working with children and adolescents with autism, respect for strengths as well as understanding of individual differences is essential, because it is through this broader understanding of the person that the therapeutic relationship is established as a tool for support and growth.

Research on the neurobiology of relationships (Badenoch, 2008; Cozolino, 2010; Porges, 2011; Siegel, 2012) has established that empathic relationships are based on a sense of connection and understanding and shared experience. At the same time, awareness of challenges is essential as well. In autism, as Grandin (2013) has described, sensory challenges can disorganize a person's thought process to the extent that it is difficult for them to identify and describe to someone else the nature of the difficulties they may be experiencing. And Badenoch (2008) has suggested that the relational information neurotypical children readily synthesize and process has to be painstakingly "assembled" by children on the spectrum. This process of discovery, communication, and integration is part of the work of therapy. Therapists need an understanding of both strengths and challenges to support this work and these relationships, and to more clearly see the person in the environment and within their network of relationships and experiences.

Chapter 6
A World Between Art and Play

The creation of a sand tray, like the creation of art, is a visual process. Yet the experience of working in the sand tray, like the process of art making, is as sensory and kinaesthetic as it is visual. The child's experience in their world emerges in the sand through the senses and through the personally symbolic figures they choose. These can be endlessly shifted until they feel and look right, without the frustration that sometimes comes in the process of getting a drawing "right." Children can move freely through the room, choosing miniature figures for play. They move the sand itself into shifting patterns.

The sand "is a material with great malleability and yet potential solidity" (McCarthy, 2007, p. 99) that allows children to explore both flexibility and containment. Play in the sand can make psychic processes visible (Zoja, 2011, p. 5). When the sand is seen as not only a sensory material but also as a rich expressive "world building" environment, building and sharing a world in the sand offers children a parallel or complementary experience to art making. Through the sand tray they can explore their experiences and understandings on a sensory, perceptual, or creative level.

Children's stories unfold in the sand as on paper or through clay. Creating a "world" in the sand both goes beyond words, and at the same time supports children in finding the words to tell the story of their world.

Sandtray/Worldplay is a flexible, multisensory child-centered way of working with children's growing edge of development (De Domenico, 2000; Richardson, 2012). Children can explore and express themselves through their play, regardless of their presenting state or their diagnosis. For children with autism, De Domenico's way of staying with the child allows expressive play to be supported through sound, movement, or a shift in the play that may include the therapist. This is similar to Greenspan and Wieder's (2009) concept of "following the child's natural interest" (p. 83) as a fundamental way to connect with the child and encourage meaningful communication. Some children may remain silent while creating their sand tray and sharing their world with

DOI: 10.4324/9781315173306-6

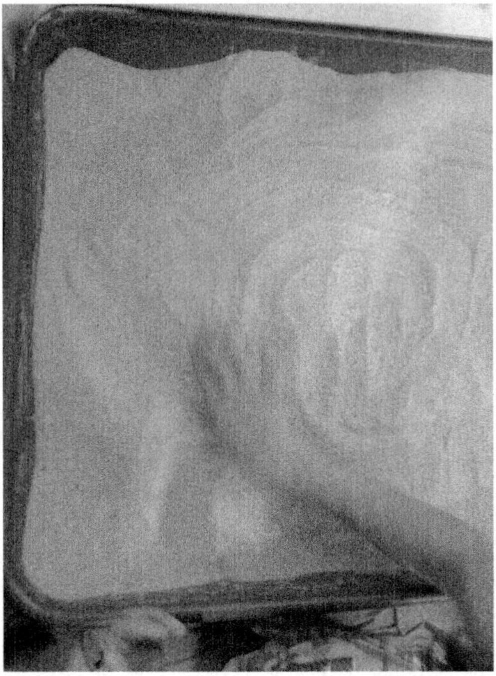

Figure 6.1 Drawing in the sand engages the senses.

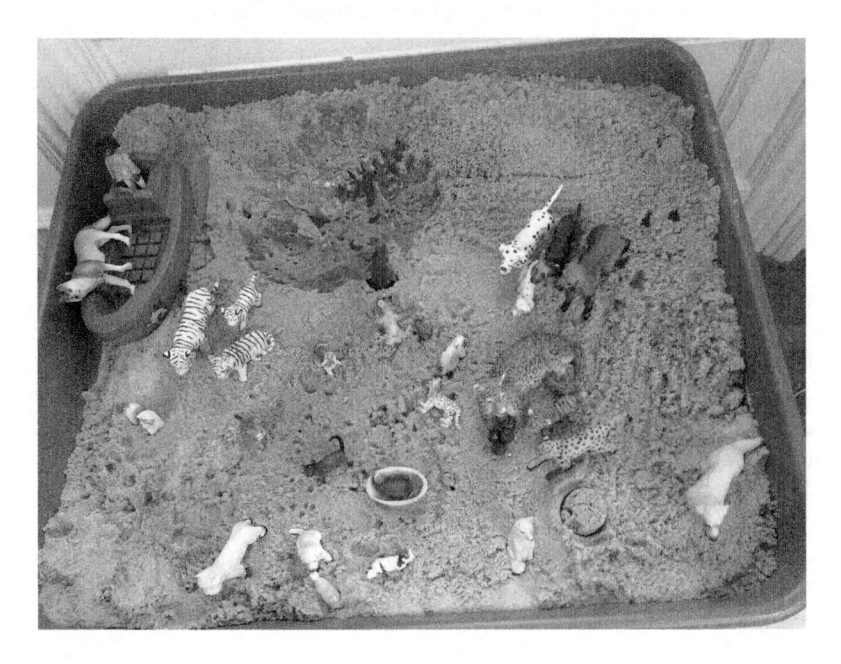

Figure 6.2 Lions, cats, and dogs in the wet sand.

the therapist. For children with autism, the emotionally charged language of play is particularly significant. Meaningful communication is encouraged by the sense of self-efficacy the child feels throughout this process. Playing in the sand may evolve into sound or movement, or into making images. Children may create figures to put in the sand or alter the figures they find to suit their vision. King Kong may be threatening, or he may transform into "a snuggly gorilla" who is welcome in the sand.

Like art making, the sand itself, and the process of building within it, is engaging on many levels: from the sensory and kinaesthetic to the creative. The sand is a material from nature. Being in contact with this malleable material can be calming and can help children to focus. Other natural materials available for play serve as "metaphorical miniatures . . . for achieving transformational healing" (Courtney, 2017, p. 112). The senses can all be engaged in the process.

Children create "living language, living symbols" (De Domenico in Richardson, 2012, p. 211) through play in the sand, as they do through making

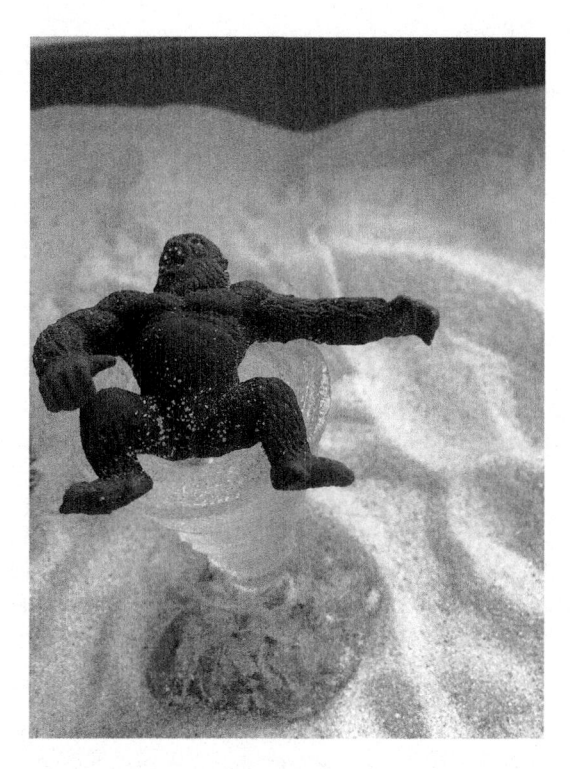

Figure 6.3 King Kong is powerful atop the tornado.

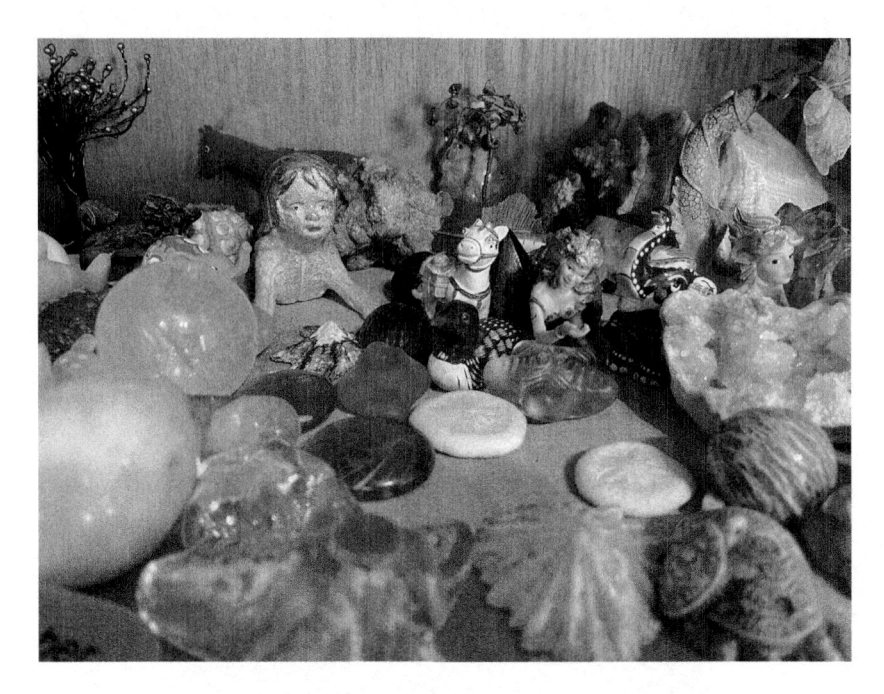

Figure 6.4 Objects from nature and magical mermaids for the sand tray.

art. The sand tray is a dynamic environment for play that can be explored on many levels, from the sensory to the symbolic. Often children enter the therapy space and immediately run their hands through the sand. Others are drawn to the shelves of figures: animals, people, magical beings, superheroes, forces of nature, and more that make up the language of images for building a world in a tray of sand.

Kestly (2014) describes the integration of these different levels, observing how in the sand, children "play simultaneously with the tactile and visual images, the bodily sensations, the implicit memories, the raw emotions, the personal memories, and the relational aspects impacting their well-being" (p. 162). Children may begin by playing in the sand and remain there for some time without adding any figures at all. Although it is a world constructed through images, it is also a world engaging the senses. One child drew a smiling face in the sand over and over, enjoying the movement of his hand through the sand which he had sprinkled with water. Then we moved together to look at smiling figures in the collections filling my shelves. He actively sought my help to identify who was smiling, and who was not. He was calm and relaxed at the end of this play, where sand was the only material he chose to use. There is a wide range of play that is possible in the sand (De Domenico, 2000)

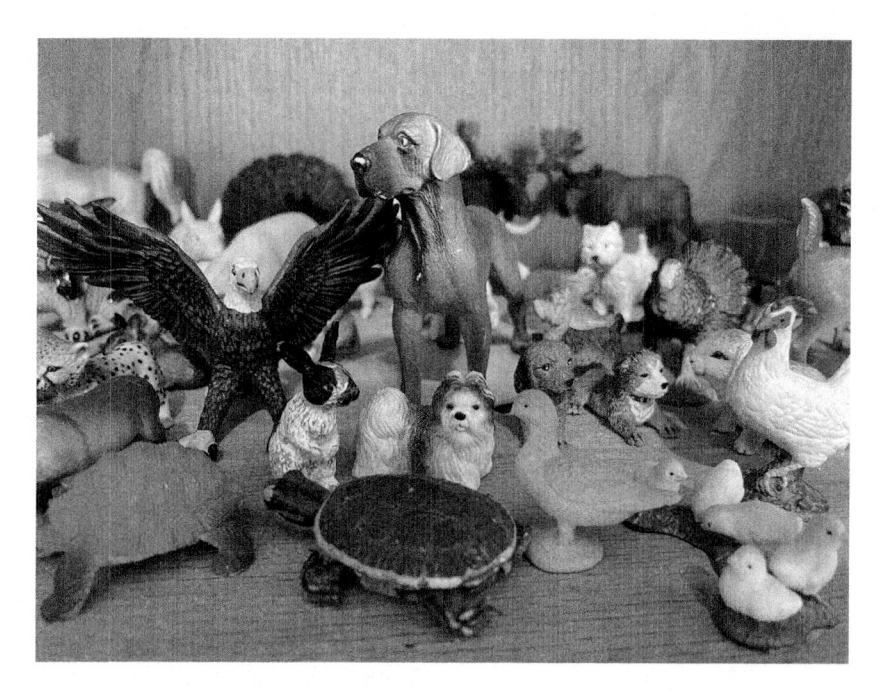

Figure 6.5 Sandtray animals.

from shifting the sand itself, to the creation of a world. There may be a drama unfolding in the sand, or an invitation to the therapist to play. As in art making, play in the sand encourages "free rhythmic use of the body in breathing, movement, and sound" (Cane, 1983, p. 37). In silence, through words, or sometimes in song, the play is created and shared.

Sandtray/Worldplay uses an "image language" (De Domenico, 2000) that is congruent with the way that some autistic people think "in pictures" (Grandin, 2006a). This visual language is made possible by the collection of natural materials, toys, and figures available for play.

It is experienced by children as valuing their interests and supporting their expression. Sometimes a verbal story emerges along with the visual one, and takes on a deeper affective dimension (Richardson, 2012). As one adolescent observed with visible relief after a challenging session, "the sand tray is a way for us to express our feelings."

While the figures for play in the sand may come from books or movies, the stories related through this play are always the children's own. Even in a story that began, as one child began, in an echo of Star Wars, "a long time ago in a far galaxy . . ." the characters arrived from the child's own universe of interests and dreams: from the world of Star Wars characters, but also from the worlds of dragons, animals, and brave children.

Many children eagerly put their hands in the sand, reaching the depths of the tray and digging, pushing, shaping, pouring, and sifting the sand through their fingers. This kinaesthetic process provides a safe base on which to build their "world" in the sand. There is the potential for calming and sensory comfort through play in the sand tray, and through the sand itself, which is the dynamic foundation for the world built by the child. Temple Grandin (2013) recollects that "When I was a child, my favorite repetitive behavior was dribbling sand through my hands over and over. I was fascinated with the shapes; each grain looked like a tiny rock. I felt like a scientist looking through a microscope" (loc. 644). McCarthy (2007) has considered the function of the sand itself for children who have neurological differences. He has observed how, for children who have difficulty moderating impulsivity, are suffering from sensory overload, or are experiencing feelings of rigidity, the sand acts as a "filter" which allows them to feel more regulated and more available for interaction.

Children sometimes articulate their sensory response to the sand, as an adolescent girl did when she looked at a world full of sea creatures and mermaids. She described one of her swimming figures as feeling "free and relaxed" (Richardson, 2009, p. 118). She made the transition between the calming process of play with the sensory properties of the sand, to telling a story. She attributed both feeling, and a parallel to her own feeling state, to a figure in her sand tray. This girl intuitively connected her sensory experience and her perception of what she had created in an emotionally resonant way. As in creating art, where both process and product are essential to the therapeutic relationship, the sand tray provides a way of being with both the creative process and the created "world" in the sand, where play and language, whether visual or verbal, are combined to make meaning (Schadler & De Domenico, 2012). Green (2012) has reflected on how play in the sand circumvents barriers with spoken language for children with autism. The innate creativity of imagining a world and a story for the figures children choose allows them to construct and share this story with or without words.

One young child made up elaborate songs for the characters he chose for his sandtray worlds. He would ask me to sing these songs with him as we looked together at what had taken place in his play, so I had to look and listen very carefully. He acknowledged my point of view as the witness to his play, and he always wanted to know what part of his song I liked the best. This was an important recognition of his perspective.

Both creating and looking back into the world they have made provide greater perspective for children. Children can explore how to create change, like the child who declared, "I'm gonna change the setting a bit . . ." to make things easier for the inhabitants of her world. Another child observed, "all the good guys are getting stuck . . . but you're stuck in a sand tray!" He then proceeded to move his little people, and the sand itself, to help provide more choices and more freedom for the inhabitants of his world, with visible relief.

Another child moved quickly from play in the sand to storytelling, as he too explored what life felt like for the people and animals in the sand. Two dogs played together in the tray, watched over by their owner, who first made sure that they would get along with a dog who was different from them. He began to narrate: "They have a wrestling match without hurting each other cause that's what puppies do . . . they keep rolling and fighting . . . and that's the point, he found a friend." Two monkey puppets then arrived on the scene, checking on the dogs, and dancing together. Before our session ended, I too was invited into the dance with the child.

The process of play and movement within the sand is about "creating living language, living symbols" (G. De Domenico, personal communication, August 5, 2006). In De Domenico's (2000) Sandtray/Worldplay model, the therapist attends carefully to the child's emerging story in the sand, in a way similar to Greenspan and Wieder's (2009) description of "following the child's natural interest" (p. 83). The sand tray is both a multi-sensory, child-centered environment, and also a process, within which a child can explore symbolic play. When a child is actively playing, communication is encouraged by the sense of self-efficacy the child feels as the builder, by the presence of the therapist, and by the therapist's interest in the child's process. Through this mindful curiosity the therapist shares in the child's world more fully. And as in art making, the process is as significant as the final image.

Sharing the world that the child has created offers the opportunity to appreciate the child's unique way of seeing and experiencing (Richardson, 2012). Badenoch (2008) suggests that, in sandtray play, the therapist "listens" to the play, "as the symbolic world unfolds into words" (p. 220). Through experiencing play alongside the child, as Malchiodi and Crenshaw (2017) explain, engagement from the therapist "frees the child to communicate" (p. 4). Sometimes a verbal story emerges alongside the play and sometimes the story is told visually through the images the child has chosen.

While children often choose the figures and images for their play silently, sometimes they may invite looking at the shelves of figures together. Choosing what they wish to play with thus becomes interactive, and begins the telling of a story as we search together for what they need. Children may turn to the therapist with questions, and these questions give a fuller understanding of the child's story. One preschooler stopped playing, and asked, without looking in my direction, "What was that noise?" I responded, "That was a really big noise!" He then turned directly to me, and I understood that there was more emotional content to the sounds he was making. He answered, "No, that was a bad guy noise." He then found helpers to join in the play. They called out, "Go away! Go away!" to the "bad guys," as he covered them up with sand. A little smurf stood up to a confrontational action figure, telling them to "get out." Even a tiny kitten joined in, bravely meowing that they needed "help." The courage of these little figures is reassuring for children, as is the knowledge that help and change are both possible. As this young boy observed, "Help means help!" We saw great growth in communication as he told stories, asked questions, and attributed motives and feelings to the animals and people in his play. He talked both for and to the creatures in the sand with an increasingly astute perception of their relationships, as he suggested to them, "you have to listen," or, when this proved impossible, reminding them that others, "need space."

Supporting children in recognizing the helpers as well as the dangers in their worlds can be done subtly, but it is important. Children sometimes identify these helpers as well as the dangers for themselves, choosing additional figures or reassuring their sandtray characters. An adolescent made a superhero ask all the people in his sand tray, "Are you sure you didn't need any help? . . . I could have helped you." In this way he was able to talk about what he himself needed to help him feel more comfortable at school. His question "Are you sure you didn't need any help?" was as useful to him as it was to his characters. He went through his mental list of all his teachers and recognized who he could go to when he was having difficulty.

Another adolescent chose to play with Batman, and this superhero declared "I can only feel happy . . . I don't have any other emotion." Along came a different figure, the angry red guy from the movie *Inside Out*, whom he introduced saying "I'm always MAD," and another who confided "I'm always SCARED." His task was then to acknowledge all of these feelings for himself, and within himself, as his characters interacted in the sand.

Younger children may not be able to have these sorts of discussions as part of the sandtray process, but they too experience a sense of mastery through their play. Some children may remain entirely silent during play in the sand, and may also have limited verbal sharing with the therapist when they have completed their sandtray world. Yet commensurate with the sense of mastery that children experience through the play, spoken language often blossoms as well. Through playing with their preferred figures, be they animals, people, or trains, children are able to create a coherent visual narrative of their thoughts and experience. A preschooler who loved big cats initially said only "lions go in sand," as he proceeded to choose every lion in the room to create an elaborate scene in the sand during his first session. His language was emerging during this time, and through his sandtray play we saw great growth in communication as he told stories, asked questions, and attributed motives and feelings to the animals and people in his play, initially with very few words. One day he thoughtfully chose a child to move among the lions, remarking, "she's not scared of lions." He then chose a cat, reassuring them that, "that's baby lions" and reminding them, "don't be afraid of a baby lion!"

His lions began to introduce themselves, coming out from where they were hiding and declaring themselves, saying, "I come from the wild jungly jungle," sharing their names, revealing their stories, and connecting with others.

A World Between Art and Play 65

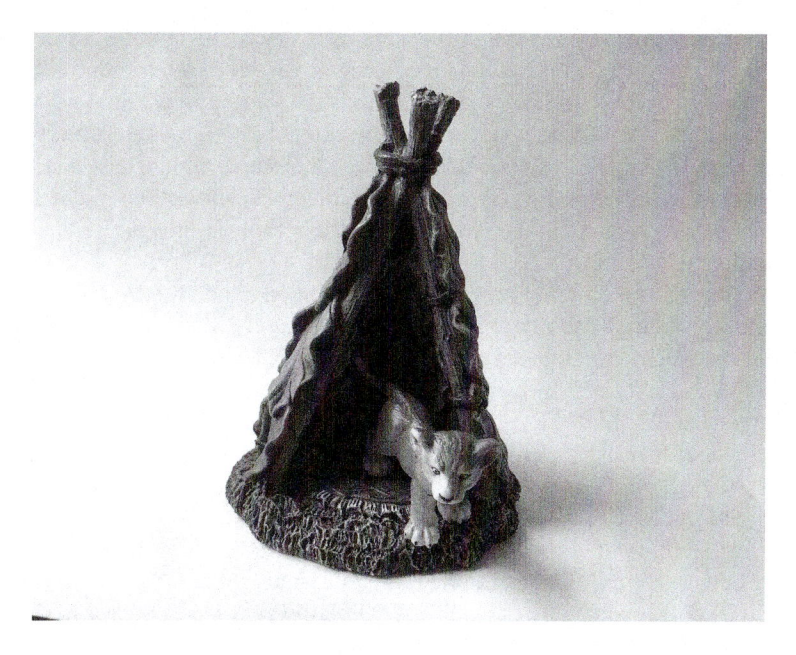

Figure 6.6 The baby lion in the "jungle hut."

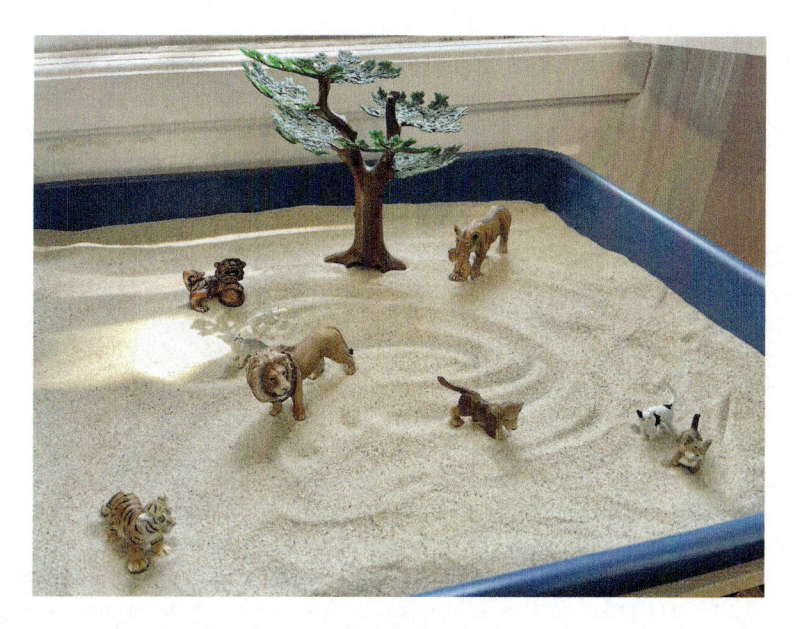

Figure 6.7 Lions, cats, and a Chinese "dragon lion."

When the lions became frightened, this child took on the role of a giant himself, stomping his feet and using his biggest voice. His lions talked to one another and thought of a strategy to stay safe, saying "I fool him," and calling out "Don't get me." He also attributed motives to a scary "goblin guy" who tried to frighten the lions, asking him "Why you did it?" The lions shared their intention to "fool" the goblin, much to the child's satisfaction. He seemed, as I was as well, fascinated by his characters' intentions and actions. He helped his animals to respond to the challenges he gave them in thoughtful and collaborative ways.

At other times, children may appear to feel stuck, and searching for alternatives to what is unfolding repetitively in the sand. This is when the therapist can suggest (as long as we are prepared to have our suggestion rejected) that there might be helpers we could find together, so that something can change. I have found that this feels similar to offering children a "third hand" in art making. Many helpers sometimes need to come until a child is ready to declare, "that's it!" A preschooler chose sea creatures for his sand tray, and remarked on who had come into his world, saying "that's a giant whale!" With great expression, and in a voice very different from his own, he loudly made a dolphin exclaim, "that's a giant whale . . . I'm going to run away!" But when other creatures swam into view, he visibly relaxed and said, "I'm so happy." He created a palpable sense of safety for the animals within his world; and he thought about what children need to be comfortable as well.

Choosing Charlie Brown to place in the sand, he introduced him to the other children in the sand tray, saying, "Hi, I'm Charlie Brown." When they ran away he cried out, "wait . . . I'm just a little boy." This story was similar to what had occurred with his animals, but his people articulated their stories, and their needs, in a different way. Charlie Brown, together with Snoopy, "his friend," said "we miss our home." He created a home for them using blocks, making sure that there were enough rooms for all. The theme of home as a comforting place was very important for this child, who had recently moved, and who was still finding his bearings in his new home. One day he chose a little house with a roof that opens. He placed it in the sand, and then experimented with putting everything scary that he could find inside, notably skeletons and huge insects. He then firmly closed the lid.

The fears he was mastering were his own. He was waking repeatedly at night and having bad dreams. Containing the skeleton made his sandtray world both dynamic and safe. At the same time, his sleep began to improve, and he experienced fewer nightmares that woke both him and his parents.

Older children may be more explicit about the fears and challenges they are trying to master. An anxious child in elementary school, who had persistent fears about her safety, called out to the animals in her sand tray, "Please gather your little ones and keep them safe." And a middle school child, actively working with fears of natural disasters, asked of each object he added to the sand,

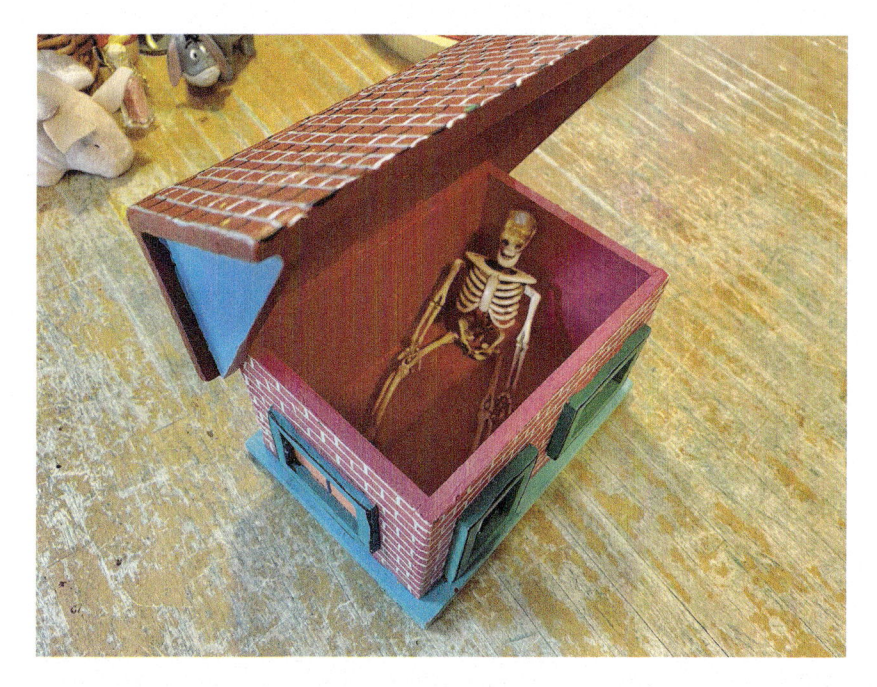

Figure 6.8 The skeleton about to be closed in the house.

"Is it okay if I put these in? . . . it's scary and creepy." When I reassured him that he could put in anything he wanted, and as much as he wanted, he added a big handful of tiny plaster skulls. I suggested that if we put these frightening things in the sand, and can see them, that can help them be less scary.

He then added what he declared was, "the most dangerous animal in the world . . . this big cat." He repeatedly stopped and checked himself during this play, taking figures out of the sand and saying "that didn't happen." With the reassurance that there was no way to make a mistake in play, he became more absorbed and animated, as a sand tornado rained down, the scary cat meowed in an earsplitting yowl, and a hobbit scrambled to safety out of the sand. He then declared, "I'm gonna change the story a bit." He began with the repetition of the storm, and the total destruction of the scene in the sand. He built up and then destroyed a city, first unleashing a tornado, and then a volcano that came and covered everything in sight with sand. Calm finally returned to this scene. He breathed slowly and deliberately as he cleared away a space that become tranquil blue water.

Children sometimes tell a complex spoken story alongside building a world in the sand. One such story explored a child's preferred activities. A challenge for him was to balance his fascination and preoccupation with online games and his desire for connection with others. As he placed his figures in the sand he narrated:

> There was a man who lived with his two cats Fluff and Buttercup. Every day he takes care of his cats. He pets them and feeds them and takes care of them. What he did while his cats were playing is he loved playing Fortnite. The cats didn't mind. They'd watch him play the game. The cats adored him and he adored his cats. They lived a happy life because they were friends. He loved playing this game but it didn't stop him from making time to play with his cats. The cats are cool little creatures who like to do things.

In the sand and through his storytelling, this child demonstrated what De Domenico terms our need "to play with others, and for others to play with us" (personal communication, May 6, 2008), which remained true for him no matter how absorbed he was tempted to become with online games. Constructing the meaningful exchanges essential to our ability to communicate and build reciprocal relationships through play in the sand also helps children to understand and build relationships within their families, schools, and communities. This child was able to reflect on his family relationships and on his relationships with the friends with whom he liked to play online games. He began to understand that there can be more balance in how he shares with others.

After a world is created, the child and the therapist are "joined together, asking questions in the world" (G. De Domenico, personal communication, May 27, 2008) and seeking to understand the connections to the child's life. Witnessing the child's choices of images and themes acknowledges their importance to the child. Exploring the world and its story together builds the therapeutic relationship, much as sharing finished art does. And sometimes, art making comes into the sand tray itself.

Despite a sandtray collection of hundreds of figures, sometimes children want, or need, to create their own images for the sand tray. One child who was fascinated by geography created "a country" in the sand, and added a hand-drawn flag to his scene of pyramids and a sphinx. It took a long time for him to arrive at this moment, as he followed the history of the "country" he had created, as it formed and reformed, with the sand "blowing away" and structures "crashing." This was a very dynamic process. He observed that neither he, nor the people in his world, were scared of the changing weather and landscape. He himself was dealing with fears of storms and their danger. In the sand tray, he was able to control and observe the changes as they unfolded. Once all was calm in the sand, and he sat and drew, our conversation moved away from geography and weather, to art itself. He looked up from the drawing he had begun, and asked me "what is art?"

While he had often experimented more briefly with the sand tray, on this day he spent a long time creating and playing. He depicted a scene inhabited by people for the first time. When he had finished, we explored his question. I suggested, "I think sometimes art can be a way for us to show what we are thinking about . . . or what we like." He smiled and nodded. We talked about the images he had just made in the sand tray and about his drawing of a flag he invented and cut out to add to his world.

When he started creating his country in the sand, he gave me a hint as to the identity of this faraway place, saying "in this city they make paper out of plants. And they use shapes for letters." I was able to guess that he was building "Egypt" in the sand; and when I shared that I had just made some paper the day before, he became really excited. I asked "would you like to do that the next time you come to see me?" He said "Yes" and then he asked, "Can I draw on it?" I explained that the paper will be wet first, and then when it gets dry, that he could draw on it. I knew that he would love this process, fascinated as he was with combining and creating. We recycled some paper for him to form into new paper and to create his own colors, shapes, and symbols, making his world his own.

Whether a child is actively drawing, painting, or playing, the therapist's interest in what the child is creating supports their process. Through mindful curiosity, the therapist shares the child's world more fully. Autistic children may start out being very directive toward the therapist, and then become more flexible, but they need to understand the therapist's intention to engage with them in this play, "just like you want me to" (Richardson, 2012, p. 211). Once their world, or their art, has been created, there is time to silently share what has been created. The focus remains on the world or the art that the child has created. Looking together, and sharing the world that the child has created, allows for appreciation of a child's unique way of seeing and experiencing their world as well as their play.

Chapter 7

Playful Art and Artful Play

An Integrative Approach to
Art and Play in Therapy

Play can be artful and art can be playful. Both open-ended play and the arts are informed by the senses and by the creative process. When we look at play developmentally, we can observe the process through which children explore and transform the "potential space" described by Winnicott (2005), thus growing into their lives and relationships through action and interaction. Children's play and art are an invitation to experience their world together with them. Whether a child is actively playing or creating, building in the sand tray, forming clay, drawing or painting, or collecting materials to create an environment, the sense of self-efficacy and self-awareness the child experiences is encouraged both by the experience itself, and by the presence of the therapist. The therapist's acknowledgment of both the process of creation, and of the finished creation, encourages the growth of relationship and communication. Working from the base of the child's strengths and using the process of creativity in therapy helps children and adolescents to reach their potential. One child, playing in the sand and creating a world that mirrored his own, said "I don't even know how I was able to do that!" The interplay between different expressive languages is a valuable tool in therapy. Sometimes children's play appears almost like a drawing in motion when it is witnessed by the therapist. As one young boy filled the doll's house with animals, he added essential things for a puppy, who already had food and a bed. He declared, "He needs love," and chose a heart from the sand tray shelves, nestling it inside the house close to the dog.

When children shift from more sensory-based and exploratory play to verbal or visual expression of heartfelt emotion, their play embodies a story and sometimes a metaphor for feelings and experiences. In the play with the doll's house, this child focused on creating safety and also explored nurturing.

Another child created an environment by filling the office floor and chairs with colored silk scarves, connecting the colors to feelings as he laid them around the room. Since, he decided, purple was "scary" and red was "sad," he helped a baby doll to move away from these frightening feelings. He experienced himself as able to create safety, as well as perceive safety. These feelings and metaphors are likely to arise out of child-centered play and art making.

DOI: 10.4324/9781315173306-7

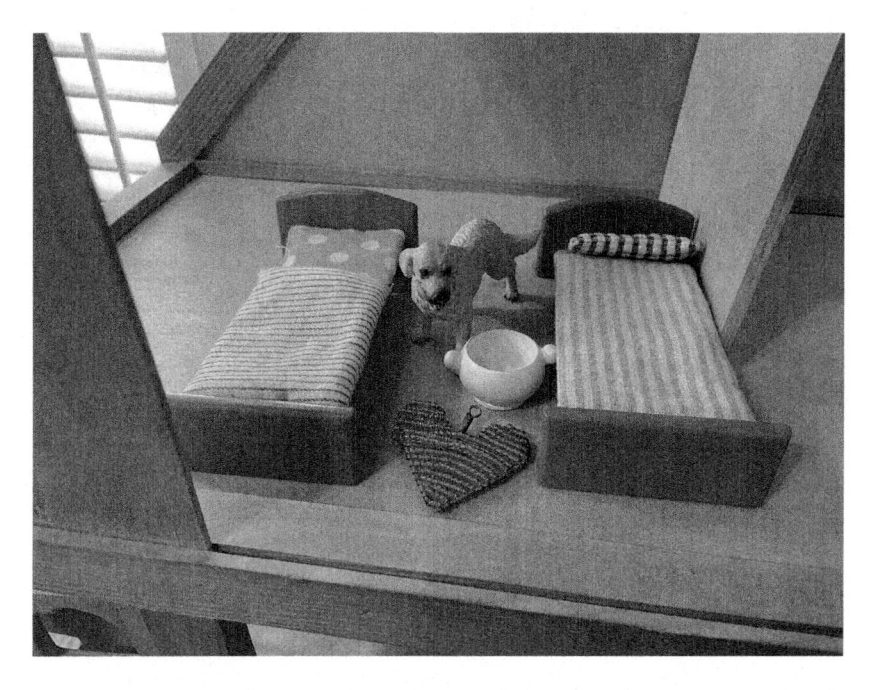

Figure 7.1 The heart in the house to comfort the dog.

But when children are feeling stuck or dysregulated, the therapist can offer structure and support. Understanding the balance of child-centered and more structured approaches in therapy is as integral as understanding the materials and processes for art and play.

Playing and art making are expressive experiences that may be nonverbal. As Schadler and De Domenico (2012) describe, the sandtray process moves "gently into language to develop a story after it is experienced on a deep level" (p. 90). Badenoch (2008) describes how, in play therapy, "both people listen . . . with their whole bodies . . . spanning both hemispheres" of the brain "as the symbolic world unfolds into words" (p. 220). Moving from art making or play, or from the world of the sand tray and back into the child's life, can help give children the capacity for greater flexibility. Porges (2011) has suggested that, "the goal of therapy is to enable clients to experience greater flexibility in the world" (p. 244). And Gil (Gil et al., 2014) suggests (p. 112) that an integrative approach supports flexibility in treatment.

While building rapport and trust with autistic children may take longer than it does with other children, these trusting relationships can be formed in therapy, and they constitute the base of successful treatment. For children with autism, a certain inflexibility stems from their greater difficulty in making generalizations, taking the perspective of another, or moving beyond narrowly defined interests or feelings of perfectionism (Richardson, 2012). As Hull (2014) has observed, in the beginning stages of therapy with children with autism, it can be hard to establish the relationship. He describes how, "some children don't talk" while "others talk incessantly" and some may be overwhelmed and thus, "bounce from toy to toy" (p. 402). Children may also be preoccupied with arranging objects or playing with fidgets that fascinate them, and move slowly into more expressive or interactive play. A combination of acknowledging the child's interest and following their lead, and intervening actively to provide an engaging experience that is shared, helps children to be more playful and interactive.

Children are often particularly fascinated by the magnets in my basket of sensory toys and fidgets. Many children could happily play with these for an entire session. Once they are ready to share the magnets with me, I cut out a little person or animal from paper, and prop it up between two powerful magnets so that it stands up. Then, I can move this figure around the table. Children love to try this, because they can feel the pull of the magnets, which are quite strong. Once we have two figures, we can create a relationship and a story with them. Sometimes children continue to elaborate, even making a backdrop for their tiny characters. Finding these sorts of expressive and dynamic ways to explore what children perceive and feel through creative, shared activity has been characterized by Henley (2018) as a "creative response," the interpersonal medium through which "challenges can be transformed into expressions" (p. 7).

Sometimes a creative response needs structure as well as support to emerge.

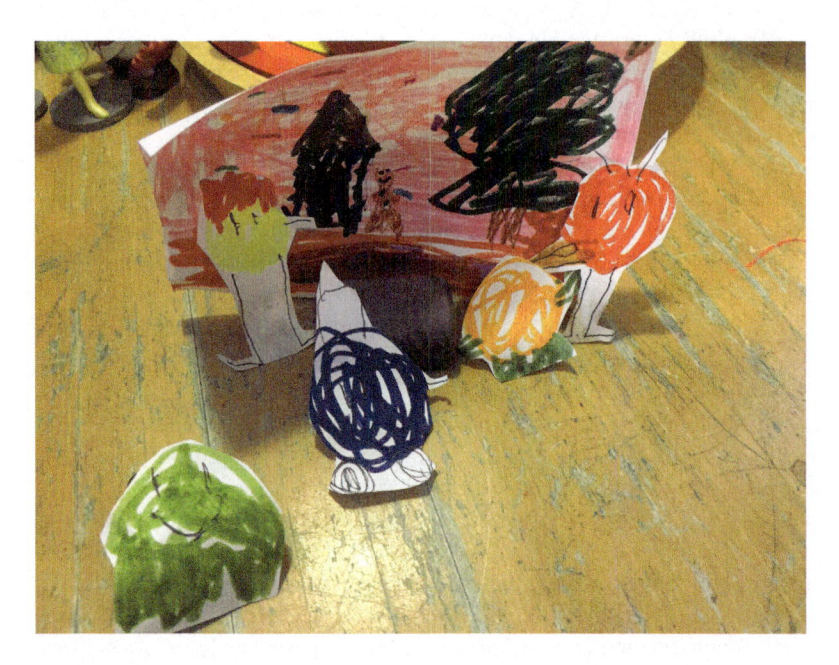

Figure 7.2 Magnetic people and their world.

When the therapist connects with the child, shared art making and play allows communicative and relational abilities to blossom. Acceptance of an autistic child's uniqueness and interests as they are expressed through art and play allow a child to feel special in a positive way. Bromfield (2010) has highlighted this "specialness" as an essential element in the success of creative approaches to therapy (p. 92).

One young child came into therapy accompanied by the observation that "he has no play skills." As Greenspan and Wieder (2009) have observed, children "who have motor or processing problems have difficulty imagining the world and thus pretending" (p. 83). However, as this boy engaged in therapy, his mother described him as "making connections" not only in his play, but in his relationships and ability to communicate (Richardson, 2012, p. 224). While he began therapy eager to "battle" with my puppets in every session, he became increasingly interested in the sand tray and the smaller figures for play in the sand. Research by Macari et al. (2021) suggests that expressive and engaging puppets "may facilitate therapeutic efforts" for autistic children through capturing their attention. For this child, the puppets held his attention and supported greater engagement in play, and in therapy. As he began to play with a greater range of puppets and other toy figures, both the powerful animals he chose to play with, and he himself, began to find resources and helpers. As he moved from the energetic and exhausting puppet battling of his early play, he searched for safe places for the animals he placed in the sand, "because they don't really like the battle" (Richardson, 2012, p. 218). He found friends for even the fiercest of dragons, declaring, "Now the other dragon will have a friend, the same kind he is!" (ibid). The dragons learned to cooperate, create safety, and to share. Another child focused on the storytelling potential of the puppets, responding to the "talking tree" that I often use in sessions to engage children, as he created a portrait of the "tree man" who regularly joined in his play.

As Bromfield (2010) suggests, therapy with autistic children and adolescents is complex. Therapy must address both the core challenges of autism and the child's emerging feelings and experiences, and support communication with them. Goals for therapy must not be targeted solely to remediating deficits (Wetherby et al., 2000), but rather must "create the types of contexts that are more responsive and conducive to communicative intentions" (p. 124). Children with autism struggle with communicating emotional experiences, and with articulating their emotional difficulties. Moreover, the impact of stressors can be exacerbated when children's perceptions of events are colored by sensory and communication challenges.

Ray et al. (2012) have pointed out the importance of nonverbal communication in Child- Centered Play Therapy for children with autism. They note the way in which the therapist follows and responds to the child's play and movements, "to communicate in nonverbal ways to increase meaningful interactions through gestures" (p. 167) and build relationship through "meaningful symbolic interaction" (ibid). In child-centered therapy the therapist meets

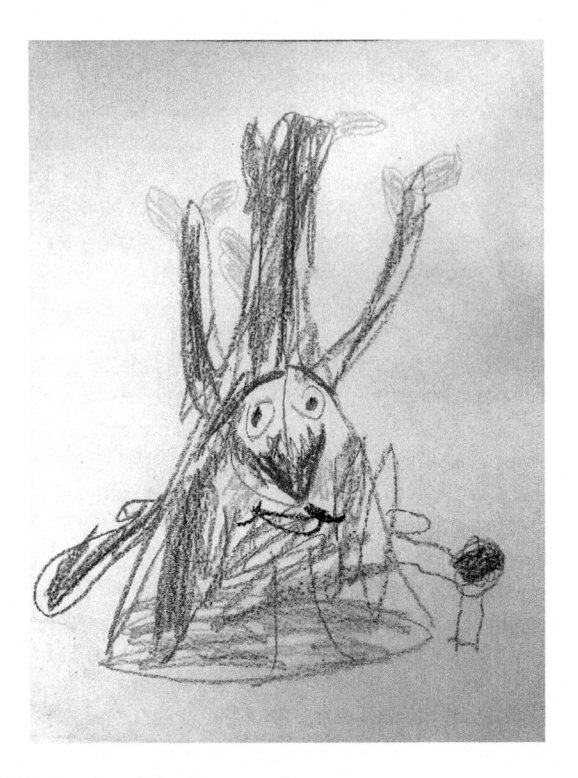

Figure 7.3 Child's drawing of the "tree man" puppet.

the child where they are. Art and play reveal the child's perception of the world and their interests. In more structured or directive art or play therapy approaches, the therapist has specific art and play based ways to engage the child and meet the child's needs as they arise.

An integrative approach allows for movement between more open-ended and more structured therapeutic interactions with children. The integration, or "blending" (Mills, 2014) is exemplified through the integration of art and play. Lara (personal communication, March 10, 2012; Lara and Bowers, 2013) has observed how children portray their inner experience through art, play, or movement without spoken language. When children are comfortable and receptive, speech and language can be stimulated both through movement and through the processes of art making and play. A flexible approach enables therapists to look more broadly at what creates change and supports communication. The therapist needs both to engage the child wherever they are, and to address the specific concerns that brought them to therapy through providing new experiences and supporting new skills.

Van Lith et al. (2017) examined best practices for art therapy with autistic children and found that being either overly directive or too loose with direction exacerbated children's communication difficulties. Similarly, while non-directive play therapy can build children's abilities in social responsiveness (Josefi & Ryan, 2004) and self-regulation, Stagnitti and Pfeifer (2017) suggest that autistic children will disengage from open-ended play if it becomes too difficult, and therefore is no longer fun. I have seen children stop short while playing, with a stricken expression, and literally say, "I don't know what to do." Grant's (2017a) AutPlay Therapy, is very clear about delineating the way in which therapists need to be aware of this balance between following the child's lead and providing direction. In his "Follow Me" approach the therapist "lets the child lead, but always gets involved with what the child is doing" (p. 49). Later in the treatment process, specific therapy goals are addressed in a more structured way. Following the child's lead, as Grant explains, allows for connection with the child and supports communication. The optimal level of support and structure from the therapist allows children to remain engaged in therapy, and to grow in their ability to play, create, and communicate.

Children can be very clear in how much structure or interaction is comfortable for them. A young boy handed me the turtle puppet that I had showed him during an earlier session. I had demonstrated, and he had experimented with, how the turtle could pop in and out of his shell if he was feeling interested and safe, or duck back inside if he was feeling uncomfortable or scared. He gave me the role of checking out potential friendships for the turtle. He introduced bugs, a bear, and a fish and these characters shared good things to eat. Although he talked little, he was able and eager to identify behaviors which were "friendly" and elicited sharing. He spontaneously suggested to the puppet characters that they "breathe and relax" when they were feeling scared, knowing that he had created a place that was safe for them. And, as he reminded me, the turtle had his shell to keep him safe.

Sometimes a bit of structure or support, such as offering a different material, a different puppet, or a musical instrument, helps a child to remain engaged in the open-ended process of play and creating. And sometimes it proves to be too much. On one occasion a child handed me a small monkey puppet, while the child squeaked away, moving with the larger "grown up" monkey puppet around the room. Following the child's lead, I too began to squeak, but was swiftly silenced. I was told, "if you use that voice, then it means that my therapist would be acting strange." On another occasion, a child and I scurried around the room together, putting out the "fire" of volcanic lava he had created, complete with his sound effects. While this child had begun the session feeling angry, he soon became engrossed in the playful process, laughing and twirling and feeling powerful. Nevertheless, he stopped playing just as we were surrounded by a pile of fiery colored scarves. Holding a huge blue cloth that was designated to be our "water" to quench the lava, he asked me, "You know this is just pretend, right?" The movement between the "pretend" world

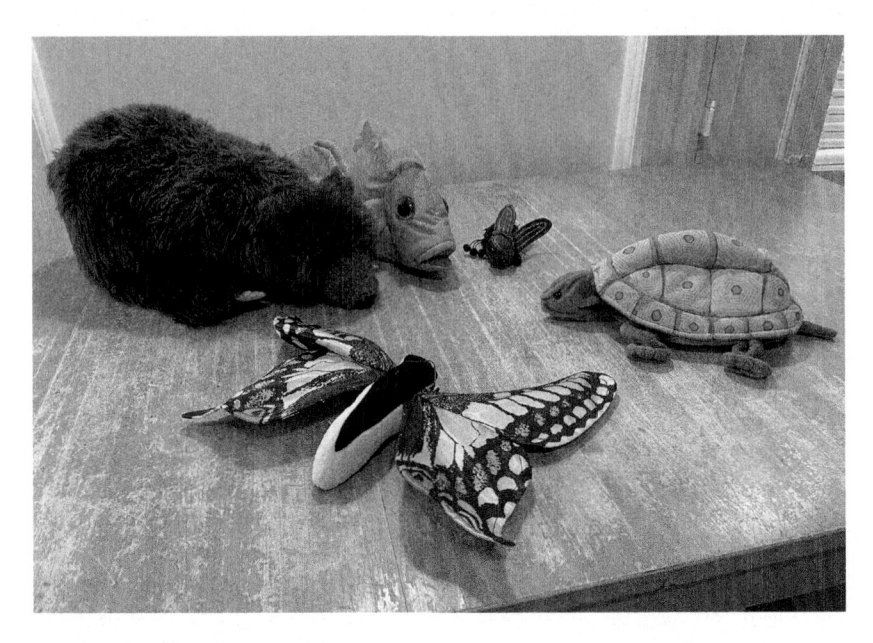

Figure 7.4 Friends for the turtle.

of play and the present moment in which the child and the therapist are connected, helps the child to play more freely, and to find the connections to their own life through play. In the sand tray, for example, children create a story, and the child and therapist then learn together about what may be taken from this world the child has created, whether there is verbal storytelling or not. While staying with the child as they play in the sand, as they create a "world," the therapist can connect with the child, attending to meaning and engaging the child's interest.

For a young girl transitioning to a new school, a sequence of sessions alternated open- ended art making with more structured experiences. This progression built toward establishing the therapeutic relationship and exploring strengths as well as challenges. In an early session, she chose to work with clay, and deftly created two seals, coaxing the clay into shape. They were, she said, a mother and a daughter seal "who like to be together on an island" which she created for them. I offered her a huge blue stretch cloth to create "water" for the seals if she wanted. When she invited her mother into the office toward the end of the session, I suggested that she and her mother could use the stretch cloth to move together, like the seals through the water, and the two climbed into the long swath of fabric together, laughing as they gracefully moved through the room.

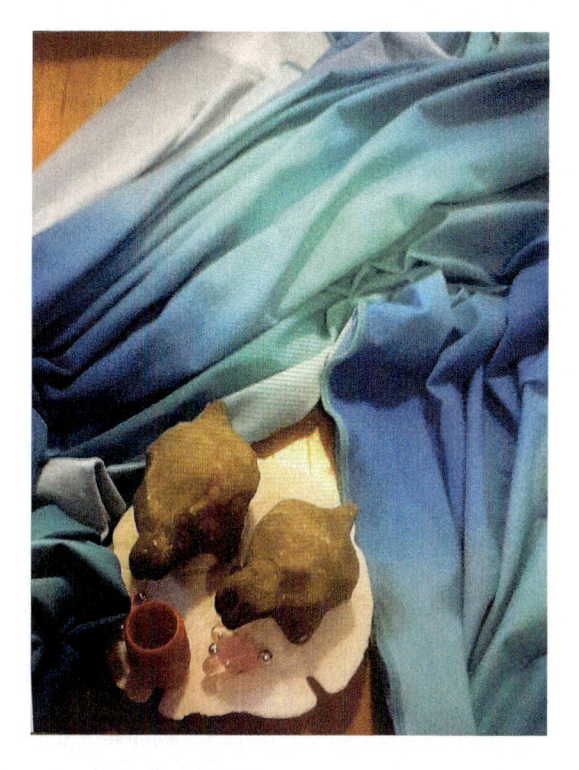

Figure 7.5 The seals and their world.

With her mother's help, we discussed strategies to help her to feel more comfortable at school. In a later session, she again reached into the bin of clay, and relaxed by kneading and rolling the material, all while talking about her day. She created a zebra first, and then a leopard, placing them together, "so they have a friend." She was able to talk about how while these animals are different from one another, they still share some of the same preferences, like playing ball together, and eating ice cream. She created everything they needed, including their favorite flavors of ice cream.

As she painted her clay figures the next week, she mused about making new friendships, and talked about the children in her new class. She talked about how the animals she created were able to understand one another. We also explored how she was feeling at school, and how much more she now understood about her new class. At the same time, she was more readily able to recognize her own strengths as they were evidenced in the treatment setting: listening, and being very observant as well as creative. She displayed a growing ability to communicate and to ask questions when she was confused, together with a wonderful sense of humor.

After initially following this child's lead in initial sessions, with specific suggestions that built on her spontaneous process of art making and play, I suggested that she create her classroom in the sand. She had talked in detail about where everyone sat in the classroom, who worked together, and how she felt about her place there. She carefully created little tables from blocks and placed everyone in the sand. As she set up the classroom, she identified the qualities of all the children and of her teacher. Creating this "classroom" helped her first to visualize the children in her own small working group, and then to consider their interactions. She thought about who was helpful, who is a "stressful" person, and who helped others. In this way, the new group became more familiar to her. With prompting from the therapist, she was able to notice her own strengths as a focused and engaged student, as well as recognizing that she could ask for help from her teacher. Creating the affectively meaningful exchanges so critical to the ability to communicate and form reciprocal relationships in therapy (Greenspan & Shanker, 2004) can support building these relationships within the family, the school, and the community.

As children engage in therapy, including the therapist in their play and sharing their art, such themes of connection, communication, and relationships may also be explored more spontaneously. When children feel connected and safe, suggest Badenoch and Bogdan (2012), "we can perhaps begin to sense that play and interpersonal connection work as a synergistic system" (p. 9). Sometimes children create this comfort for themselves before they even begin to play or to make art. One child set up the therapist's smiling cloud figure, and turned a bop bag into a person, sitting them beside him and saying, "They will watch us while we draw." And another child positioned the doll she had brought into our session cozily in her lap, gently guiding her hand across her drawing as she drew with a crayon.

Prizant (2015) suggests that the feeling of dysregulation should be seen as a defining characteristic of autism. While many children—with or without autism—enter therapy struggling with anxiety and self-doubt or presenting with challenging behaviors, autistic children's underlying feelings of discomfort may be more acute and persistent. Mills (2014) has noted how while sensory imbalances may not appear to be a challenge for all children, "we have found that they do play a consistently pivotal role in determining how the child copes with the presenting problem" (p. 79). This is particularly true for children with autism. When children are feeling comfortable on a sensory level, they are able to do the work they have come to therapy to do.

One child talked about "how big kids need to feel little," when they need a rest, as they cozily settled into a chair with a silk blanket and a stuffed horse. A young child who brought a favorite stuffed animal into a session demonstrated how the process of connecting through the senses works. Sitting his little stuffed bird on my art table, he reached into a basket of fidgets and pulled out the "magic window," with colors that flow across a screen when it is gently turned. He sat the bird right in front of it, and then proceeded to make the

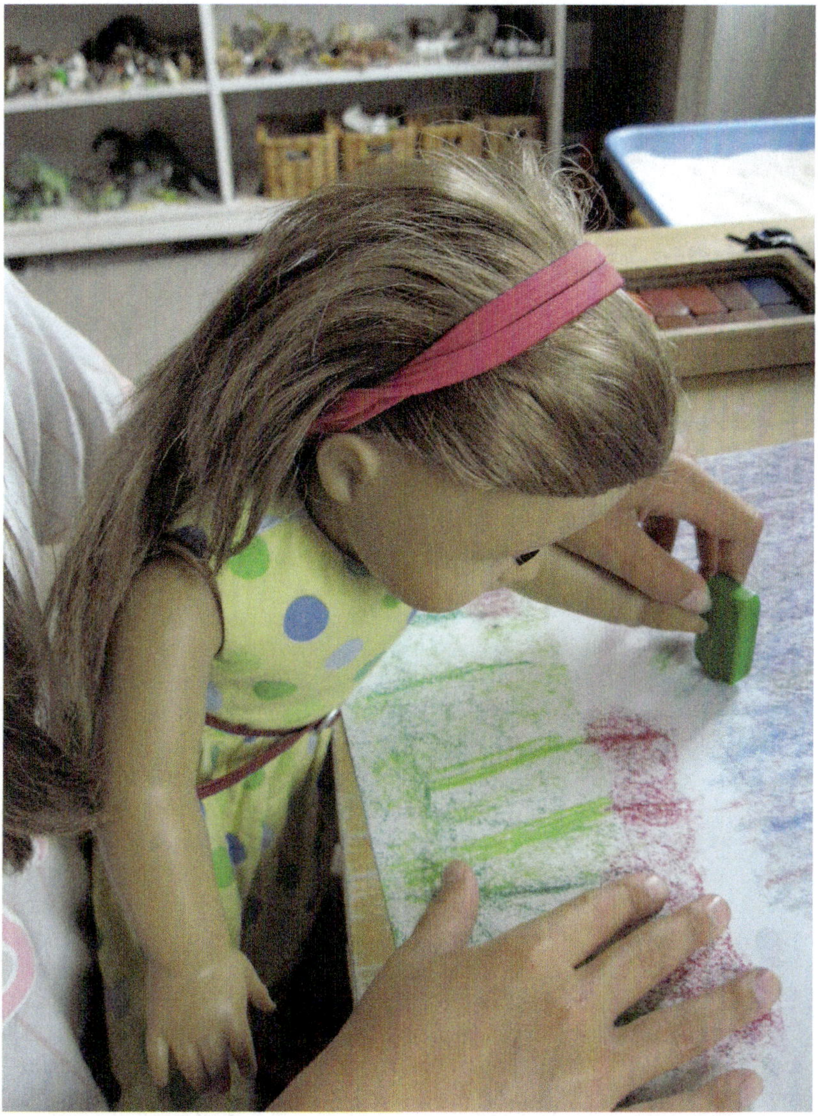

Figure 7.6 The drawing doll.

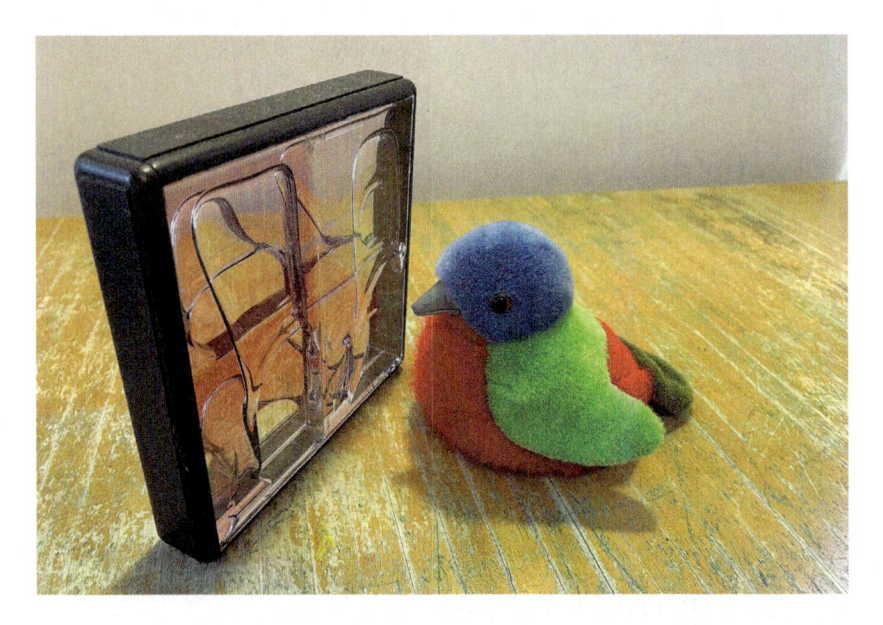

Figure 7.7 The bird in front of the magic window.

colors move and swirl. Next, the boy and the bird investigated my collection of stress balls and kaleidoscopes, and then he pronounced that he was ready to play. He had just conducted a therapy session for his little bird.

Children can also be helped to engage through their senses and to share a story, with or without words, through rhythm (Daniel & Trevarthen, 2017). A young girl talked about using her senses and movement to cope with the stressors of school. She had the idea that she could gently move her "head shoulders knees and toes," to feel more comfortable, and realized that she could always have access to this source of comfort. Sometimes children's rhythm and movement is more dramatic. When an older child was feeling very stressed, he immediately flopped into a big chair. He then curled up in a ball, quickly wriggling himself behind the chair. The chair banged into the floor, again and again. I handed him a small drum. He played, first loudly, and then more quietly. When it was quiet, I slid some paper and markers in his direction. This usually painstakingly accurate and observant young artist filled the paper with seemingly random scribbles, pressing so hard that the paper ripped. Slowly he emerged from behind the chair. I reassured him that he had done just what he had come here to do: to understand how he was feeling, to communicate that, and to find a way to feel more comfortable. Children need plenty of time for sensory experiences to feel comfortable and connected.

Research has found that openness, flexibility, reciprocity, and the opportunity for shared experiences meaningful to the child are critical elements of play therapy approaches for children and adolescents with autism (Greenspan & Wieder, 2009; Mastrangelo, 2009; Myers, 2009; Wetherby & Prizant, 2000). Play therapy then facilitates social interaction, joint attention, and emotional regulation (Hillman, 2018).

In art therapy, a similar balance of flexibility and structure supports therapy goals for children with autism (Van Lith et al., 2017). Among the helpful practices Van Lith and others (2017) have identified were: maintaining a consistent routine to begin each session, consistent explanations of instructions for using materials or processes, and awareness of the importance of transitions. This survey further suggested that acceptance of a child's communication style helps to support a successful therapeutic relationship.

I have had many children benefit from a timetable which we created together to outline the flow of a session. This helps them to understand how much time we would spend together, and where we would each be making choices for what we would do during this time. Not all children need this amount of structure, and some experience it as somewhat intrusive, but all children need to have their communicative efforts accepted and supported. Essential to a successful integration of art and play based approaches is acceptance of a child's overtures of communication and scaffolding this communication through the processes and materials for art and play. Prizant (2015) has characterized how successful therapists "adapt to the situation rather than stubbornly sticking to a fixed agenda or a prescribed program or plan that does not reflect the needs of the individual it is destined to help" (p. 141). Schuler and Wolfberg (2000) similarly point out that:

> The practitioner's dilemma is one of balance. Although more directive adult-structured approaches may be overly controlling, more child-centered approaches that attempt to acknowledge the child's state of mind and try to follow its lead are often too subtle to draw in the child's attention. One of the challenges in the design of effective intervention thus lies in the creation of child-centered structures that are neither too loose nor too rigid.
>
> (p. 257)

Some children need a very clear, repeated structure within each session to find this balance. I have made little books with children, outlining the sequence of our sessions. This is particularly helpful for children who become so absorbed in their special interests that they have trouble communicating about them or sharing them. With structure, the child knows that they will be able to freely draw, paint, or play out their interests as well as sharing their art and play with the therapist.

Other children and adolescents need structure to gain a sense of perspective about their worries or fears. While children can draw or play out in the sand the various escalating components of their worries, it can also be of help to create a calibrated "worry meter" for talking about worries. Importantly, this sort of organization helps to identify when worries need to be shared so they do not escalate. One adolescent created a timeline of feelings, so he could see the times when he began to feel uncomfortable or unsupported, particularly at school. I wanted to help him recognize the need to take a break or to seek help before his distress escalated. He created a model of the physical classroom itself on my art table, using figures from the sand tray, blocks, and cut out figures that he had made. Literally looking into this creation engaged him on a bodily level, helping him to explore his felt experience before moving into the more abstract process of creating his timeline and solving the problem of when he needs help.

While nondirective play therapy can build children's abilities in social responsiveness (Josefi & Ryan, 2004) and self-regulation, children sometimes seek more direction from the therapist. Older children in particular may "not know what to do next" after being swept along by initial enthusiasm for choosing what to play with and surrounding themselves with the materials for play. Younger children may not be able to take the next step in playing with what they have chosen.

One day, a story that a child was playing out with puppets did not feel right to him. We talked about how it is okay for a story to not be "perfect" and work out exactly as he planned, with every prop for the action arranged flawlessly. We explored whether playing could be more spontaneous and still be fun. His play then moved into a theatrically less elaborate, but emotionally more resonant, interaction between two puppets. The theme of their different expectations for what they were doing together was quite similar to our evolving interaction with one another. While the child wanted to create an elaborate puppet show that was ready for prime time, I, as the therapist, hoped that he could use the puppets to tell a story that would be satisfying to him, and connected to his own life. I also wanted him to relax and to have fun.

The little dragon puppet watched the adult dragon breathe fire. The little puppet—just like this young boy—was able to manage his frustration at not being able to perform this powerful magic, and to come up with a way to get attention that was playful but appropriate. We talked about how playing can be a good way to "work things out." Sometimes this "working out" can happen together with family members. Another child used the puppets to practice moderating demands that felt "in your face" to his mother when he asked for things. They played with the puppets together; and while they experimented with different proximity to one another, they were each more relaxed in this playful interaction than they had been in their frustrating discussions of their problem.

Playfulness can serve as a way to defuse anxiety, creating space to work on problem solving. Children are also able to use creating as a coping strategy. Henley (2018) describes a child who "by making things by hand . . . could

Playful Art and Artful Play 83

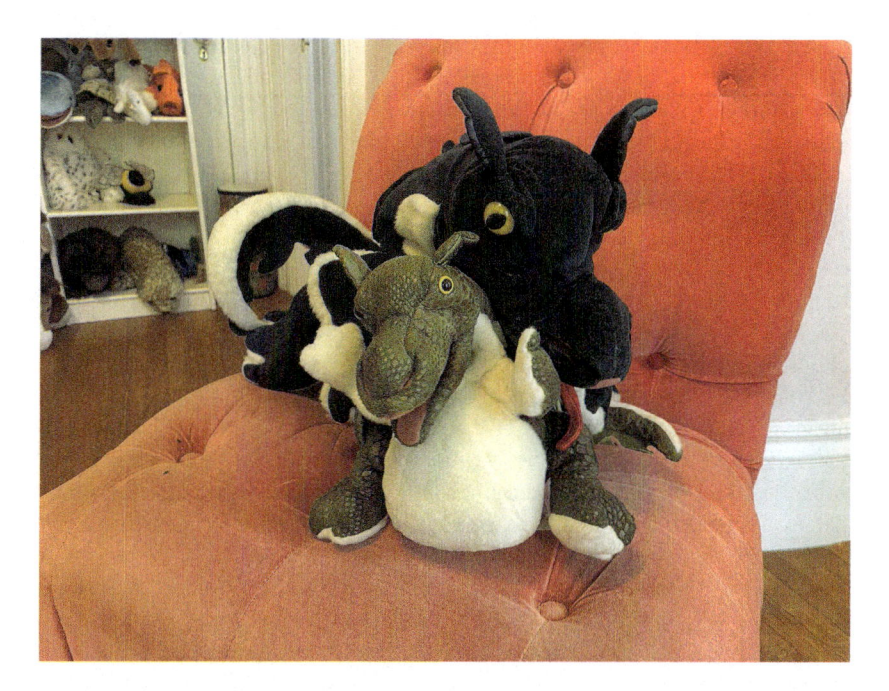

Figure 7.8 Large and small dragons.

desensitize disturbing realities" (p. 49). Children are often aware of how this process works for them, and they adopt creative expression as a resource. As one middle school child decided, when peers at school make him upset, "I can draw a cartoon of them." He created a series of artist trading cards for "things I care about," working with great attention to detail in a process that was calming and focusing for him. He then had some images to carry with him and enjoy or share, since they were so small and portable.

Support and structure from the therapist both helps children to grow in their ability to play and create, and to remain engaged in the therapeutic relationship. Sometimes this deeper engagement comes from the therapist's response to the child's actions or artwork. One young child who had been struggling with outbursts of anger when he felt uncomfortable, came into the room and began to play an angelic sounding melody on a xylophone. After quietly listening, I told him how calm and happy his music made me feel, and he smiled. Later in the session, when he chose figures to play with in the doll's house, he wanted me to participate in this play. I took one of the figures, the bright red "anger" figure from the film *Inside Out*, and saw an opportunity to see if he could work this musical magic on this enraged little guy. While returning to music making was not his own idea, he was willing to try. I made the figure jump up and down on the art table. The child again played his "relaxing" music, and I made the figure slow down and calm down. The child's play continued with lots of sharing and nurturing among the sandtray characters he had chosen. These were both new themes in his play, and he had begun to learn skills for greater self-regulation through play and creative experience.

Sometimes children enjoy planning sessions. One child, proud of being "the leader" chose a relaxation story (Khalsa, 1998) that we had used together to share with his sibling and mother. Everyone relaxed on cushions or on the floor, and calmly followed the imagery of the story he had chosen to read. Khalsa's story describes, "a very soft white cloud" that has come down, "to take you for a ride." The story continues, "Feel yourself going up, up, up, into the beautiful blue sky . . . breathe gently as you travel through the sky . . . ahead of you is a rainbow" (p. 91). The children and their mother then sensed the feeling of the rainbow colors washing over them, and the peace and comfort of gently returning to the earth. Everyone chose a rainbow-colored scarf that made them feel safe and comfortable. Our young leader spontaneously said that the color he had chosen made him think "of love."

Steele and Malchiodi (2012) suggest that what makes a process we use in therapy feel safe in this way is how "it is presented and applied" (p. 94). And Van der Kolk (in Steele & Malchiodi, 2012) describes how "safety, predictability and fun are essential for the establishment of the capacity to observe what is going on, put it into a larger context and initiate physiological and motoric self-regulation" (p. 95). This child felt calm and regulated, and was able to share his comfort and creativity with his family.

Yoga, Relaxation, and Regulation in Therapy

When introducing an approach that is both new and structured, such as yoga relaxation, it is important to first tune in to the child. Khalsa (2016) has observed that a new experience can be introduced successfully when the therapist or teacher first observes, "what moves them—what they are interested in" (p. 122), and then uses creativity to introduce a new activity that feels connected somehow to what children are doing. Introducing yoga and relaxation into sessions, as Pliske and Balboa (2019) suggest, through integrating "yoga, play therapy, and neuroscience philosophies, can help bring a comprehensive treatment approach to children's mental health issues" (p. 81).

Some children with autism may feel anxious or unfocused and therefore physically uncomfortable within themselves or within the therapeutic space. It can be challenging to bring awareness to the child of where they are in space, and to what they are doing with their bodies. Goldberg (2013) says "often children just don't know where their hands are" (p. 69), and they may not feel in control. During new experiences, whether with movement, breathing, or relaxation, the therapist observes the child's response, being especially mindful of tension or anxiety that arises. If a child sits more securely, or moves more comfortably, beginning to appear more settled, then they are probably ready to try something new. Sometimes children need to experience what they are feeling, even if it is dysregulation, before they are ready to make a change (A. Morgan, personal communication, July 16, 2017).

While children feel both movement and breath, they are able to see movement. Using props for breathing helps children to be observant, and to see if something changes when they breathe. They can blow a feather, gently, and then more vigorously to see what their breath can do. Breathing brings a sense of rhythm. For children who don't have a good sense of rhythm with either their bodies or their thoughts, this will affect their breath as well. They can feel their breath more with their eyes closed, and they can gain awareness of their breath by seeing what it can do. After one child blew on a feather, he thoughtfully said: "I have more energy blowing the end than blowing the fuzzy part. That makes me calm." Another young child told me, "I breathe when I feel nervous." We explored how he breathed at this time when he felt comfortable, and not nervous, using a sphere ball to see the expansive process of breathing in and out. We also used our own hands to create a sphere while we were breathing. After we made "the earth" with our arms, at my suggestion, the child wanted us to make "the moon" as we breathed in and out. Their breath is a tool that is always with children. When they have more conscious awareness of how breathing can be calming or energizing, they have greater self-awareness and self- regulation. The awareness of their breath, and of where they feel things in their body are similar to the internal awareness that is integral to EMDR, which also helps children to focus on uncomfortable situations and sensations and move toward comfort. When children do something as simple as touching their palms together, or when they try putting a hand on their belly and one on their heart, this is both comforting and orienting.

For children with neurological challenges, there is a tendency to function in a state of stress. Emotions and physical sensations are both involved in this process. Children with autism may be especially susceptible to stress because of differences in their autonomic nervous systems, according to Porges (2011), giving rise to self-soothing calming behaviors. He suggests that, "since there is now documentation that children with autism have lower levels of vagal tone and do not efficiently regulate it . . . yoga could be an efficient portal to improve this system" (in Goldberg, 2013, p. 66).

Similar to blowing on a feather to see the breath, listening to the sound of the ocean in a shell can help children to focus, but also to observe themselves. These activities can be either calming or energizing. A sleepy child in my office has often engaged after focusing in this way. And a very active child, in turn, has often calmed down while listening to the sound of the ocean, or learning to blow on a feather so gently that only the soft, tiny edges of the feather stir with the breath. Since yoga addresses sensory processing challenges, and can be focusing and energizing, as well as calming, feeling movement through yoga helps children to focus and experience calm. Goldberg (2013) has observed how, for many autistic children:

> Thoughts, feelings, sensations bombard them continually, increasing their levels of stress and forcing them into fight or flight . . . Regulating the breathing, practicing quiet relaxation and turning inward for mindfulness practices are ways to introduce children with special needs to the process of stilling the mind.
>
> (p. 76)

Balance in the Body and in the Brain

When children present with challenging behaviors, "usually the answer . . . is that they are experiencing some degree of emotional dysregulation" (Prizant, 2015, p. 18). It is this dynamic that brings children and adolescents with autism in to therapy. Prizant (2015) suggests that feelings related to dysregulation can help to explain children's behavior in a more meaningful way. Guest and Ohrt (2018) surveyed autistic children treated in play therapy, and found that the "differences in perception of everyday events" (p. 157) for children on the autism spectrum exacerbates the impact of stressors, and may even render events traumatic to the child. As 63% of children with autism (Guest & Ohrt, 2018, p. 157) struggle with the ability to communicate emotional struggles or experiences, Guest and Ohrt suggest that flexibility and responsiveness to the child in treatment are fundamental elements of effective therapy. Even when traumatic experience has taken place, these researchers found that while building rapport and trust took longer than with many children without autism, that a trusting relationship was both possible and formed the base for successful treatment. Expressive approaches to therapy can effectively support children "with limited language skills or less developed experiencing skills" (Schadler & De Domenico, 2012, p. 90) and can work with their creativity.

Understanding the neurological aspects of autism is essential to understanding how art and play engage children in therapy. While it is easy to observe when children are dysregulated, it is not always easy to delineate the experiences leading to this state, nor to find the way back to greater balance. Children's behavior may appear chaotic and confused—enough so that they are incapable of responding calmly to an interaction, an activity, or a communication from others. It can be helpful to see children's challenges, whether they be meltdowns or withdrawals, as a manifestation of a lack of integration on a neurological and physiological level (Siegel & Bryson, 2012; Badenoch & Bogdan, 2012). As Prizant (2015) suggests, challenging behaviors may stem from an effort to gain control of overwhelming outside stimuli and of themselves.

Children are able to use art making for self-regulation and regaining balance, as well as for expression and communication, as Malchiodi and Crenshaw (2017) have observed. Cane (1983) discussed how art making begins with "free rhythmic use of the body in breathing, movement, and sound" (p. 37). Helping children to feel regulated through movement allows them to connect and communicate more fully. Therapists have a responsibility to help children become more regulated and more resilient so that they do not become as stressed and distressed; but they have an equal responsibility to build better supports for children in all the contexts of their lives. Steele and Malchiodi (2012) have posed questions that are very important for children on the autism spectrum in this regard. "What," they ask, "if we never ask a child what really gets him going, but also never ask what really calms him down? . . . How can we support his efforts to self-regulate?" (p. 84). Once comfort has been established in the therapeutic setting and relationship, then it is possible to address "what gets children going": the meltdowns, anxiety, mood, or social challenges, or the disruptions in a child's life that have brought them in to therapy. A successful "language" for therapy is one that allows children to experience and share their emotions and make sense of their experiences.

The very materials used in play or art making are powerful because they can physically connect emotion and experience. Kestly (2014) suggests how even "just catching sight of the resources for play begins to touch the parts of our brain, mostly in the right hemisphere, that hold our unresolved painful or frightening experiences" (p. 524). And for children with autism, says Robert Jason Grant (2014), playing "offers the ability to communicate inner processes and emotions without using verbal communication and provides awareness properties to help put words to otherwise unidentified issues" (p. 16). Children's need for sensory comfort and the developmental need for rhythmical regulation, as Kestly (2014) has discussed, means that "play props that provide this kind of sensory input are important" (p. 101). Such props could include sensory fidgets, kaleidoscopes, cushions, and expanding spheres of all sizes, that as Kestly (2014) says, "can be easily manipulated to synchronize with the rhythm of our breathing" (p. 101). Other materials, such as silk scarves, stretch cloths, and parachutes, can be used in movement or as props for both transforming the space itself and creating a safe space for the child. The materials, environment, and space become increasingly expressive as the child learns to feel comfortable in the space and with the materials.

Children's neurobiology affects their ability to feel regulated and connected to others. Siegel (Siegel & Bryson, 2012) suggests that the initial challenge with any children who are experiencing distress and a lack of integration is to help them "become better regulated so they can use their whole brain in a coordinated way" (p. 6). Prizant (2015) explains how this sort of integration, which enables us both to self-regulate and connect with others, can easily break down for children and adolescents with autism, as their neurological makeup makes them particularly vulnerable to stressors. Prizant stresses the importance of understanding both the sensory needs and the processing behind meltdowns or repetitive behaviors. Other people, he notes, can provide a positive "presence and proximity" (p. 24) that supports emotional regulation. One role of the therapist is to provide this presence. He explains how:

> For children on the spectrum the experience of integration can support greater self-understanding when parents, therapists, and teachers encourage them to use all of their capacities and move beyond feeling "stuck" within inflexible patterns of thought or behavior, such as melting down or rigid adherence to order.
>
> (p. 24)

The likelihood of misperceiving a situation as unsafe or overwhelming is more likely, and receptivity can be more challenging, for children with autism. Generally, in typically developing children the awareness of and response to risk will be somewhat accurate, that is, their understanding of risk "matches their gut response to danger" as Porges (2011) characterizes this process (p. 13). Children, including children with autism, can be in a receptive state for new learning as long as their environment and relationships support openness. When children are unable to use their brain in an integrated fashion, such receptivity to relationships and experiences is not present. Porges (2011) further explains how "areas in the temporal cortex that are assumed to inhibit flight, fight, or freeze reactions are not activated in people with autism . . . who have difficulty with social engagement" (p. 16). Helping children to move from the closed off state of reactivity to a receptive state produces a more positive felt experience. Children then become more open to what others are sharing with them.

When children are feeling strong emotions, they need help to comprehend and communicate about their experience. This is an integrative process of being comfortable with, and understanding, emotions and sensations. And if "we want to prepare kids to participate as healthy individuals in a relationship," suggests Siegel (Siegel & Bryson, 2012), "we need to create within them an open, receptive state instead of a closed, reactive one" (p. 129). In my office I have a stuffed figure of a smiling brain, and one of a heart. Children are curious about why they are there. But they are able to both match them to their own bodies, a process that usually leads to laughter, and to consider what it means to use their hearts and their minds together, connecting their thoughts, experiences, and emotions.

Helping children to become more flexible in their behavior and interactions means nurturing and supporting both neurological integration and the child's own self-awareness. For children and adolescents with autism, the mechanics of bridging the left and right hemispheres, which is a function of the corpus collosum, can be more difficult. Lara (2016) has observed both how difficult it is for children with autism to integrate horizontally, and how active movement supports this integration, helping both sides of the brain to work together in a more flexible fashion.

Calming strong reactions and impulses, and accessing emotions are valuable self-regulatory abilities that are supported by both vertical and horizontal integration in the brain. Horizontal integration allows for left brain logical processes to integrate well with right brain emotions. Vertical integration, or the ability to use the higher level brain function to thoughtfully consider behaviors and actions, similarly needs to coordinate with lower brain functions concerned with visceral reactions, which for children with autism may be extreme. Both types of integration, as Siegel (Siegel & Bryson, 2012) notes, give children greater control "over their emotions and their body" (p. 40) as the result of a free flow between the lower and higher areas of the brain. Badenoch (2008) has noted how this integrated functioning is what supports both children's thought processes and their relationships.

Dealing with emotions, as Prizant (2015) states in the brilliantly titled, "How Not to Teach Emotions," elicits both cognitive and physiological responses from children, since we all both "reflect on how we are feeling and why" and "also experience emotions in our body" (p. 127) and through our senses. Often children with autism are taught to identify emotions in a way that is static and scripted rather than dynamic and intrinsic to the child's felt experience. Cognition and emotion must work together (Prizant, 2015) to understand such nonverbal communications as facial expressions and gestures in a meaningful way.

I sometimes model the changeable nature of emotions for children by using clay. Since the "language" of clay is so fluid, it can be quickly altered and as quickly changed when it does not feel right. While children are working with clay I sometimes make an animal figure, a person, or a little face myself, and these are there to interact with what the child has made, giving us an opportunity to explore relationships.

Putting a little visage on the end of a clay tool makes a very simple and changeable "stick puppet" that can be used to explore feelings. Despite the simplicity of this figure, children are always curious, and sometimes captivated by the smiling face. This can be altered easily, on the other side of the figure, to a "sad" or concerned looking face. Finally, with a zigzag edge tool, I create a face with a large mouth and teeth that children usually identify as "mad."

The wonderful thing about our play with these little figures is not that there is change in the feeling state portrayed, but that this change is spontaneously identified by children. They can quickly turn a figure around or even obliterate it if it is scary or not to their liking. And if, for example, a "mad" face is not mad enough, they can take over from the therapist, or create their own figure to exaggerate the expression even more. Such "meaningful manipulation" of clay, suggest Hass-Cohen and Findley (2015), "involves controlled voluntary movement, a function of the motor system that increases cognitive functions" (p. 225) and builds awareness of emotion and the ability to communicate about emotion through art. Such simple and playful interactions invite children to

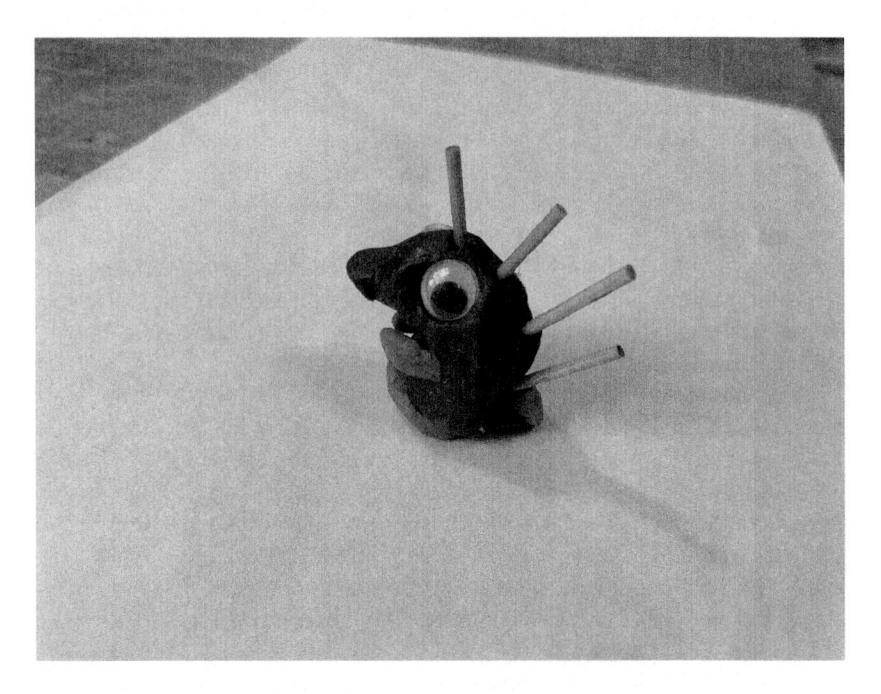

Figure 7.9 The therapist's "Baby Godzilla," a figure to join in play.

create their own faces or figures, and to connect feelings with their creations. King (2016) has similarly suggested that creating portraits engages the motor neuron system and supports interpersonal connection (p. 83). The simplicity of what the therapist creates in these sorts of shared clay or drawing experiences is deliberate, as this can be reassuring to even the most perfectionistic of children. Having their therapist create something simple diminishes potential feelings of being overwhelmed, or feeling what they are creating is not good enough.

Clay is an unstructured and sometimes overwhelming material that sometimes gives a sense of being out of control rather than one of welcome freedom. Thus even in the simplest creation and interaction, therapists must support children's willingness to "put trust into your hands," as Rhyne (1984, p. 125) has said of working with clay. In this way, therapists help children to engage with, and to learn from, the material as well as from the image, and use both to tell their stories.

A "sense of story" as Prizant (2015) calls the fundamental ability to construct a personal narrative, brings comfort and supports communication. For autistic children and adolescents, the bilateral integration Badenoch (2008) has described helps them to be aware of feelings and communicate ideas. Sharing a story or image through play, or through art, allows a child to use the safety of the therapy setting to understand events that may have been distressing to them, and to find supports that lead to change. Siegel (2012) has characterized this process as a dance of attuned communication with the child.

Understanding the specific neurobiology of autism, and the importance of integration in working with all children, helps us to construct, together with children, individually meaningful pathways toward communication and relationship building. Chapman (2014) discusses how art making involves the literal integration of the sensory and nonverbal neural pathways in the brain along with the left-hemisphere verbal pathways. Kestly (2014) suggests that play is a valuable avenue for assessing, as well as building, integration and wholeness. The process of using play and art in therapy provides many opportunities to observe children and assess their needs, as well as to support their growth. Access to richer visual expression and spoken language may come first through movement, music, and play. Working with responsive and flexible materials can encourage flexibility in the child, and exploration of new materials can lead to increased expression.

Kossak (2015) suggests that the arts literally move us to "tune in and feel sensations and emotions" (p. 7) in a rhythmical fashion. Research further indicates that body-based and "whole brain" approaches strengthen the communication between the hemispheres of the brain, effectively "waking up the brain," in Lara's (2016) description, to fuller communication and connection. Kestly (2014) suggests that, while this process is difficult to document empirically, play allows us "to be in touch with aspects of experience that language can't reach, and the resources of the right hemisphere in discovering new ways of being and behaving in the midst of the freedom of play" (p. 174). Richer expression and language may come first through art, movement, music, and play. Working with responsive and flexible materials and processes encourages flexibility in the child, encouraging the building of relationships, creative expression, and communication. While the child's materials may be simple, the process is profound.

When children are feeling dysregulated, they may be both very active and very unfocused. It is possible to see this focus shift within the session. One child consciously put what he termed "opposite elements" in a sand tray he created, describing water as calming and fire as active and exciting. His mother and I had discussed how readily he himself moved from being excited, and in an essentially positive state, into dysregulation that then presents as depressed mood or anger. Now he was noticing these feelings shift in the opposite direction, and gaining a greater sense of control.

The medium of the sand itself possesses an infinite capacity for change and repair. Children sometimes notice how playing in the sand connects them with nature. Another child came to his session having been at the beach earlier in the day, and remarked on how the sand in the tray was like the sand at the beach. He found that running it over his hands made him feel comfortable, just like being at the beach. As he wondered about the origin of the sand, he seemed connected to nature while playing in the sand tray. He appeared to feel relaxed and regulated, far away from his computer and the games that both fascinated him and made him tense.

Sifting, blowing, and shifting the sand can be as calming or energizing as children need it to be. Children observe these shifts in the sand in their play. One child who rained sand down on the trees in the tray, and then blew it around (carefully, so as not to breathe it in) reflected on how much the landscape he had created had changed. "Think of all the things . . . that have changed," he said. For a child who has difficulty with changes and with letting go, this was a comforting way for him to explore the active process of change as he himself controlled the speed of change. He was able to think about things in his life that change, begin, and end. In the sand, he observed, "you can always go back," as it is possible to go back and remember the things that you have done, as well as to imagine with pleasure "the things you would like to do."

Chapter 8
Trusting the Process in Autism

The neurological and sensory challenges of autism can make it difficult to access the calm state essential for exploring new experiences. Changes in their lives or routines often bring children and adolescents to therapy in an anxious state. This is exacerbated by difficulty in understanding the intentions and behaviors of others, and the absence of the comfort level established by a fundamental felt sense of safety. As Carley (in Prizant, 2015) explains, for a person on the autism spectrum, "The opposite of anxiety isn't calm, it's trust" (p. 73).

While exploring new experiences, suggests Grandin (2017), "a child has to be stretched just outside his/her comfort zone." She suggests that adults be aware of the ways that individual children need support to try new experiences. Addressing sensory challenges helps children to explore something new. Sounds, for example, Grandin observes, "are better tolerated when the child initiates them." While I often encourage children to try using simple instruments, there is always a much wider range of expression, and a more reciprocal process when I follow their lead. For example, I have a very engaging ball maze where the balls strike xylophone bars, and this is very popular with children, who sometimes use it early in a session while they are exploring and getting comfortable in the room. When children have started to play with sound and movement, then I am able to take out a xylophone and join in with the sounds they are making, so we can make music together. Grandin (in Prizant, 2015) has explained how her sensory sensitivities provoke fear to such an extent that, she has said, "My primary emotion is, and always has been, fear" (p. 79). She has raised a related question that therapists must address in treatment, asking, "How do things go from scary to interesting?" (Grandin, 2017). As McNiff (2015) explains, "everyone carries an inherent license to create" (p. 1). This is as true for children and adolescents with autism as for any children or adolescents. But first, they need to experience a sense of safety and comfort with materials and with the creative and playful process of therapy. A sense of safety and comfort is the ground for building the therapeutic relationship. And it is this sense of safety that enables movement in both physical space and relationships.

DOI: 10.4324/9781315173306-8

McNiff's (2015) fundamental concept of "trusting the process" in art making and therapy suggests that one way to become comfortable with the process of art making is through kinaesthetic experience. As McNiff (2015) explains, these "familiar motions and forms are always connected to our individual and natural ways of expressing ourselves" (p. 19). He describes young children's painting as a whole bodily expression, and suggests that when we create together, we are using our bodies as much as our materials. Lowenfeld (1975) observed how, when children show active physical movement in their images, they can become more attuned to their sensory, movement-based experience. Children can capture this sense of movement through color, shape, and rhythm as well as through the image itself. And children enter into the art making process more fully when they are comfortable and oriented in physical space. One day a child took my hand while I was holding a paintbrush, dipped it in paint, and began to move it across a large piece of paper. She really pushed the brush around, creating strong strokes of paint. She then let me help hold the brush in her hand. Together we experimented in spattering paint, as well as making more deliberate marks together. When she began to paint on her own, her marks flowed in a relaxed rhythm. We found an equilibrium of working together, until she painted "the end" on our large shared painting.

For children with autism, Grant (2017a) has found, it is important to engage the process of play. Playfulness is foundational to therapy with children, whether the child and therapist are drawing, making music, moving, or actively playing together. And yet, as Grant has observed, metaphorical play, or pretend play, can be challenging for children on the autism spectrum. Prizant (2015) describes how autism can be understood as "a disability of trust" (p. 73). He explains how people with autism "are unusually vulnerable to everyday emotional and physiological challenges" (p. 18) and thus they experience greater levels of discomfort, confusion, and anxiety. Thus, the initial challenges therapists face are helping children and adolescents with autism to experience the world as more comfortable, understandable, and engaging, and to experience the therapist as someone they can trust.

Children with autism can't always trust their bodies that fully. Both sensory and motor planning challenges make this process difficult for them. So while familiar repetitive motions, such as flapping, may help to create a calmer state or express enthusiasm, moving freely into the process of art making and out of their comfort zone can be a challenge. Not all children are able to move freely, or to create freely; and yet all children have a need to move, to connect, and to create.

Porges (2011) takes an essentially optimistic perspective on the communication and relationship challenges of autism, as he assumes that "many of the features of the depressed social engagement system observed in ASD may be reversed through an understanding of how the nervous system, via neuroception, responds to cues of safety" (p. 3). In the therapy setting, we support this process through the creation of a safe space and a safe relationship.

Moving, playing, and art making all take place in space. Porges (2011) feels that the therapist's challenge is to help build comfort "in both physical and psychological space until the client feels safe" (p. 113). Physical and sensory comfort are an important foundation for whatever expressive and relational experiences are shared in therapy. Malchiodi (2020) has described how one foundational way to build this sense of comfort and self-regulation is through the expressive arts. She explains the ways in which using "creative strategies" (p. 167) can support the process of self-regulation through recognizing felt responses to emotions of sensory experiences in a safe environment. While she is not referring specifically to autism, this is an important concept for working with children and adolescents with autism; since they need the experience of becoming "effective self-regulators who can sustain calm and restful alertness when they are anxious or fearful . . . and more quickly adapt" (p. 167).

Our bodies are a rich source of information about our experiences and emotions. In fact, as Siegel (Siegel & Bryson, 2012) describes, "the flow of energy and information from the body up into our brain stem, into our limbic region, and then up into the cortex, changes our bodily states, our emotional states, and our thoughts" (p. 59). The felt meaning of an experience becomes known through the influence of the lower brain and the body, and the knowledge gained from the body may then be integrated into understanding, awareness, and action. For children with autism, increased integration between left brain and right brain can also build flexibility. Current perspectives recognize the biologically based connections between the brain and the behaviors that make up the diagnosis of autism. The neurologist and researcher Martha Herbert (2012) notes that autism impacts the entire body as well as the mind and brain. Miller et al. (2015, p. 153) have discussed how "process-based," relational multisensory interventions help children to form connections and become more regulated. For one adolescent girl, working with wet on wet watercolor was a new sensory experience that supported regulation. As she stroked the paint onto wet paper, she watched the color flow, and repeatedly said, "I love this. I love the way it feels" (Richardson, 2009). She put this image in her room and used it as a focus for calming.

Creating imagery in art therapy "exists at the intersection of mind and body," according to Hass-Cohen and Findlay (2015, p. 21). They discuss "creative embodiment" as a guiding principle of their neurologically based approach to art therapy practice, noting that movement during art making, "directly contribute(s) to developmental, emotional, and symbolic values" of art (p. 46). They also suggest that children with neurologically based conditions such as autism may benefit from the sensory and motor organization needed to create art, as much as from the expressive dimensions of art making (p. 62). For children on the autism spectrum, integrative and personally meaningful experiences with art can be a doorway to connection, communication, and growth.

Malchiodi (2020), while not referring to children with autism, explains how embodied art therapy approaches, such as bilateral drawing, work as a means of self-regulation as well as a means of mark making:

> Making marks or gestures on paper with both hands simultaneously also creates an attention shift away from the distressing sensations in the body to a different, action-oriented and self-empowered focus. It capitalizes on the embodied, self-soothing experiences originally observed by Cane almost seven decades ago and takes advantage of the power of "drawing on both sides" to alter one's own internal rhythms for self-regulation and well-being.
>
> (p. 180)

Engaging with the dynamic kinaesthetic experience of art making helps children move forward through the developmental process of communicating through and about their images. Making art can change children's physical state because they are moving and breathing while they make, and then respond to, their marks on paper, or their shapes made of clay. Hass-Cohen and Findley (2015), suggest that "echoing, and imitating client's hand gestures" (p. 234) is as possible in a 3- dimensional medium such as clay as it is in drawing. Mirroring, like drawing, gives an opportunity to try new movements and to connect with another through a shared, embodied experience. The child and the therapist are together within what Trevarthen (2017) calls "the rhythms of relating" (p. 32). Through this process, the therapist, as Kestly (2014) describes, focuses on the "rhythmical" (p. 95) needs of the child as well as their relational needs. Meeting these needs helps children to trust the process in making art and engaging in relationships.

When children engage in art making in a way that is both free and focused, they feel calmer and more connected, and readier to communicate, with or without words. When they are not comfortable with this process, we can borrow from dance therapy, and try mirroring gestures with the hands in space, rather than drawing and leaving the mark of the gesture on paper. Dance therapists Athanasiou and Karkou (2017) describe how this process worked for one young child: "Just standing with him by the window and mirroring his light and quick hand movements helped them to connect" (p. 272). I have seen children run away from the art table, uncomfortable with drawing, but then respond to making gestures in space with me.

Therapists must be careful and responsive observers, as well as being fully engaged with the child. They observe the child's art making process, as well as their images, with what Rubin (2005) has called "a third eye" (p. 93). The third eye is a keenly developed awareness both of the child, and of art. As Rubin suggests, "in art or play children can do the impossible . . . they can gain symbolic access" to the world with all its intensity, challenges, and wonders (p. 26). Providing this access to expression for children with autism engages their interests and preferences, as well as addressing their needs and challenges. When trust builds in the process, the therapeutic goals of enhancing flexibility, encouraging creativity, and supporting meaningful communication are facilitated. Greenspan (Greenspan & Shanker, 2004) discusses how:

> we engage in pleasurable emotional interactions containing more and more novelty and surprise, gradually accentuated, so that they feel secure experimenting with new emotional exchanges . . . as they become more creative, they also become more capable of making inferences and engaging in higher level abstract thinking because these also depend on generating new ideas.
>
> (p. 222)

I encourage children to see themselves as active participants in making choices, creating art, playing, and communicating. They can be helped to move from exploring the environment and materials to creating with them. Through working with and exploring the process of art making, children can begin to see themselves as creators. Henley (2018) has observed how, for many children with autism, "the arts become a creative outlet and preferred personal voice—one that is critical for meaningful self expression and communication with the outer world" (p. 9). I have often heard children use the words creation or creativity when they have been absorbed in making art. Young children may say, "I want to create something with clay" and adolescents reflect more deeply on their relationship with the creative process. As an adolescent girl who loved to paint reminded me, "I know my way around my creativity."

With her permission, I shared one of her paintings with a group of art therapy students. One of the students felt moved to paint her own response to this watercolor beach scene with its beautiful light and flowing color. The student then described how:

> This is another . . . view of a beach looking towards the sunset . . . This image is also very relaxing and soothing to watch. I felt at peace while creating this art piece. I love how this image resembles a still time that will never come and go.
>
> (Richardson, 2009, p. 104)

This is the communicative and relational potential of children's art.

Chapter 9

Clay, Play, and Connection

Children may dive into my bucket of clay in an initial therapy session. One child, after quickly making sure the clay felt okay in his hands, created a table full of shapes and figures. He then played what he called "excited music" on a xylophone. He quickly returned to take a look at what he had created, and then decided that he would like to come back to see me the following week. Another child wanted to put the kinetic sand from a small tray on his face during an initial session. I encouraged him to try making a clay print of his face instead, to avoid getting the fine and clinging sand in his eyes and nose. While he was uncertain about the coolness of the clay, and wondered whether it would stick to his face, he gave this a try and then said, "I love clay!" The sensory experiences of using these different materials seemed to give these children a greater sense of control as well as pleasure, as they became visibly more comfortable and less anxious in a new setting and a new relationship. Sometimes, as children begin to create images from clay, moving beyond spontaneously exploring how it feels and what it can do, they need support to retain their sense of pleasurable exploration along with their growing sense of mastery. A young child who initially experimented with sensory materials, including fluffy, snow-like floof from which he began to create simple faces and snow man shaped figures in session after session decided at last that he was ready to use clay. From this more resistive and responsive material, he created images that would stand and not crumble. Carefully building a base and rolling and stretching forms that reached upward he fashioned a forest, with tiny figures—two worry dolls—walking through the trees, like the brave children in a fairy tale he enjoyed.

An older child arrived feeling very excited and carrying two wrestlers. He declared, "I want to make an action figure!" He demonstrated the moves wrestlers do with my child-sized, purple stuffed Meebie. After much flipping of clay tools and playing with juggling balls, we talked about what he wanted to create: a figure that would never break. He was ready to try working with polymer clay, which is difficult to soften and demanding to shape, but which has a wide range of colors and more strength when finished. He had used more easily manipulated soft plasticene before, and this was more responsive to the

Clay, Play, and Connection 99

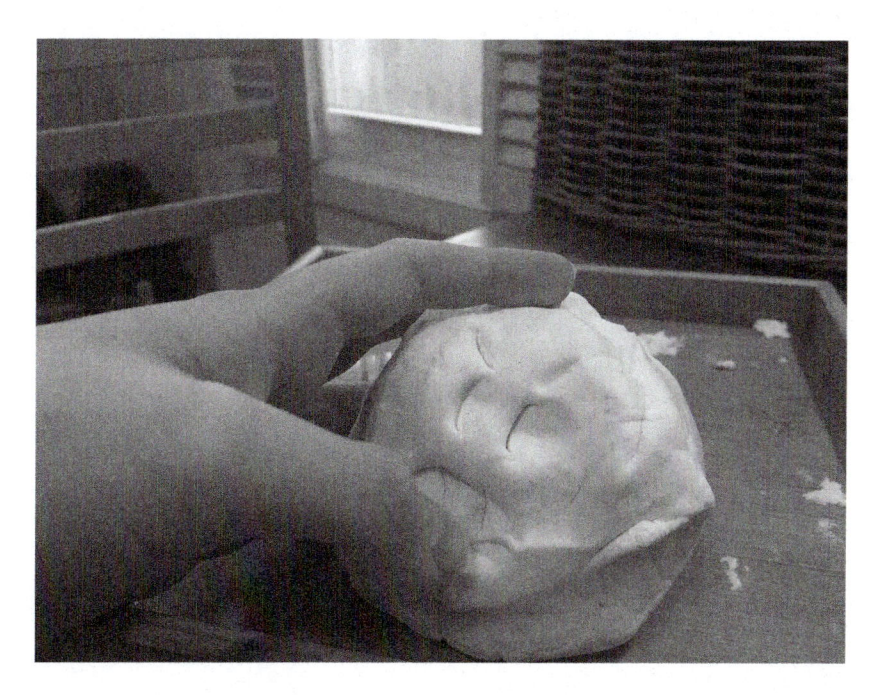

Figure 9.1 A face made of floof.

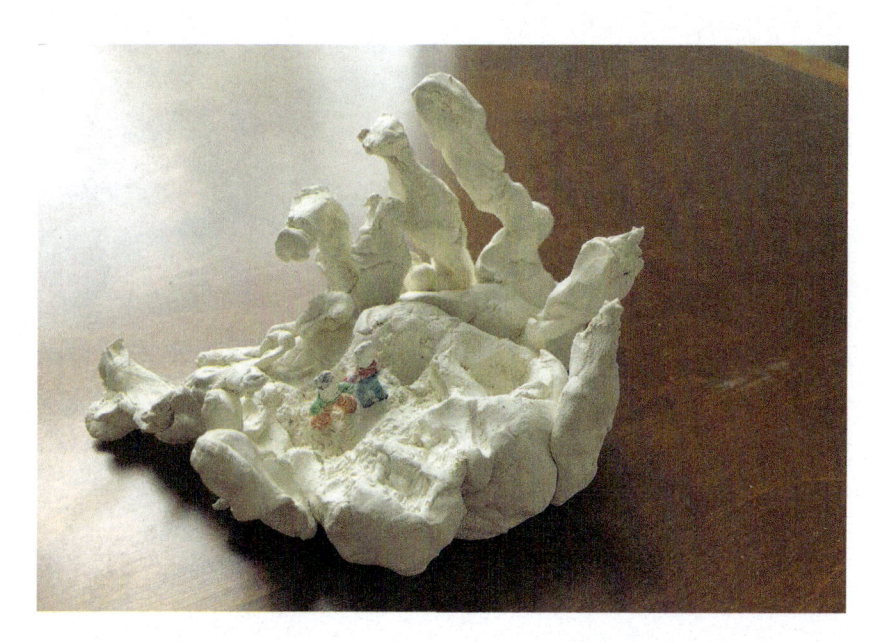

Figure 9.2 Walking in the clay forest.

gestures of his hands; and he was fascinated when I reminded him that he had used clay at our first meeting to make a simple "snowman." Now he was very focused on creating the face and the right expression for his action figure. He repeatedly checked to make sure a smiling mouth would be visible. He made more than one attempt to create these expressive features, without giving up, moderating his sometimes impulsive behavior. This child, who was often distracted and frustrated, was motivated to create.

Martin (2009) discusses how the shift to creating an image in three-dimensional space is challenging for children; and that while two-dimensional work is both cleaner and less of a sensory challenge, the clay figures children create can help them to engage in "symbolic or pretend play" (p. 90). McNiff (1998) has noted that, "clay is an excellent medium for experimenting with the way shapes emerge from the unknown . . . what appears to be random movement has a purpose in the process of transformation" (p. 30).

A "grammar" of materials, as the educators of Reggio Emilia have conceptualized this process, arises through exploration. The beginning grammar of clay, for example, might include snakes, balls, squiggles, and flowery curving forms that embody the child's physical exploration and energy. These shapes can also be altered and recombined. Working with the visual language of clay, children's "tangible expression through the eyes, ears and hands . . .

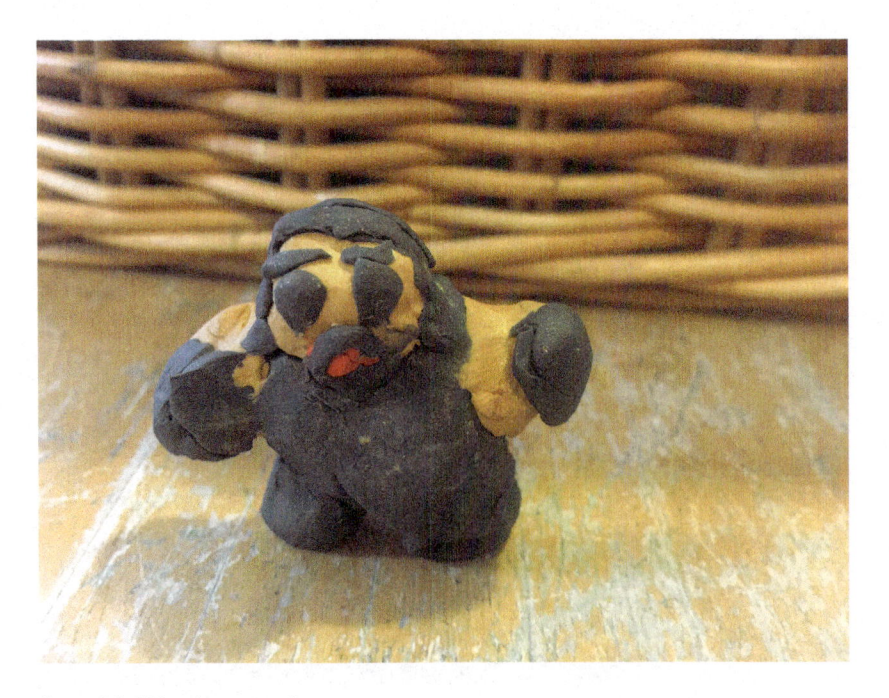

Figure 9.3 Wrestler action figure.

are capable of simultaneously constructing and feeling emotion," as Vecchi (2010) has observed (p. 12). A more complex grammar of expression helps a child to create more expressive work. This child moved from making a very simple "snowman" at our first meeting, recognizable more by its name than by its form, to a more developed and individual image.

Clay, with its malleable nature, literally embodies children's physical gestures and body language. Grandin (2015) has explained that engaging in flexible art making processes such as shaping clay are like "visual yoga," engaging the body, mind, and senses. The bodily flow that takes place through the experience of touching the clay can be absorbing and restorative. Even without creating an image (Elbrecht, 2018) an imprint can be made on the clay, and this record of the child's gesture and movement reflects change. Sensory-based, "pre-art" activities (Henley, 2018, p. 27) such as rolling or even throwing clay, as Henley describes sharing with a nonverbal and sometimes violent child, can provide a way to create a relationship. Clay is a "provocative medium," as Elbrecht (2012) describes this material, and it may not be an optimal choice for a particular child, or at a particular time. The ability to destroy the work that has just been created is ever present, and can be significant. Yet with some children, it is difficult to persuade them not to squash their figures before they have even finished them. When a child is supported through this frustration and impulsivity, a positive internal shift can happen. A child who had been throwing and breaking things at home was able to preserve his clay. He then painted this clay work, expressed his liking for the clay itself, and said, "I'm an artist." When children can find closure or satisfaction in an activity, anger and frustration begin to dissipate. Kramer's (1979) metaphor of the therapist's supportive "third hand" is especially significant when working with clay, since three-dimensional pieces need a strong structure and support to stand rather than collapsing. Children often need modeling from the therapist, and assistance to work through challenges in three dimensions. While it is satisfying for children to experiment with kinaesthetic processes like squeezing, rolling, or pounding clay, an encouraging invitation from the therapist can help move the art making from a sensory and visual activity to a shared emotional narrative and process. This "invitation" need not be a directive from the therapist, but can be a subtle shift as the therapist engages with both the child and with the materials (Richardson, 2016).

As gestures are repeated and refined, a story becomes visible through the movement and the form of the clay. When children collect and consolidate the shapes and forms they create, they make images to tell their stories. In this way, the clay becomes expressive. The movement of the child's hands and body are the means of telling their story.

Not all clay is alike, as children often point out. Sometimes the finished form seems to be the most important thing to the child, and sometimes there is a stronger sense of urgency involved in feeling and seeing the movement of the clay itself. One child described how, "this clay"—soft plasticene—works better than natural clay "because you can keep changing it and changing it." Some children value a more clearly defined form—perhaps one they can paint; and they are willing to work with the effort needed to shape natural clay. Other children may choose to work hard with a more resistive material to create a permanent figure they can save. All clay figures inhabit space, and their creation incorporates movement. As the clay moves toward its completed form, the image the child has made sometimes becomes an object for play. The improvised choreography between figures made by the child, or by the child and the therapist together, tell a story. Clay figures both embody sensations and evoke feelings.

The sensory stimulation and kinaesthetic nature of working with clay provide a rich experience for children who engage with this material. Hass-Cohen and Findley (2015) describe how: "clay inherently pulls us into a broad sensory experience that involves movement, muscles, sensation, touch, sight, and smell," (p. 214) and how this sensory experience with the material "serves as a gateway to mental representations of memories, perceptions, and emotions" (p. 207). The gestural nature of working with clay can be mirrored from child to therapist, or from therapist to child, initiating an interactive and relational

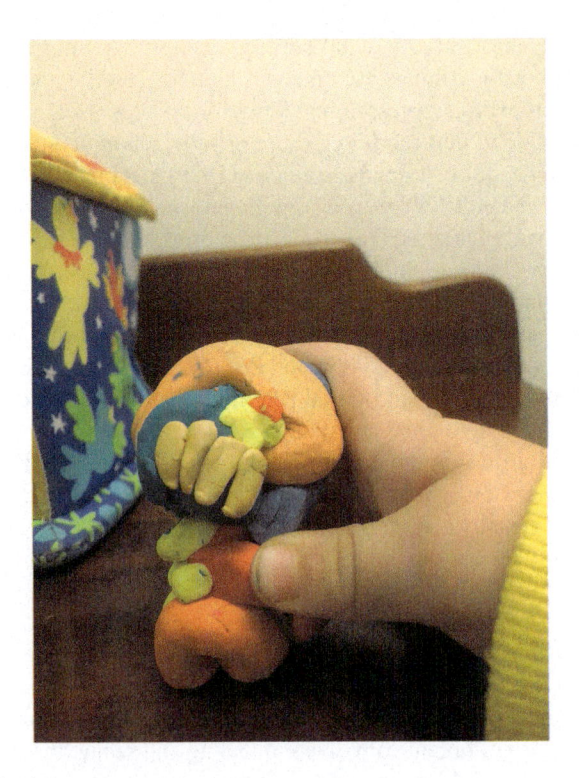

Figure 9.4 Plasticene creature.

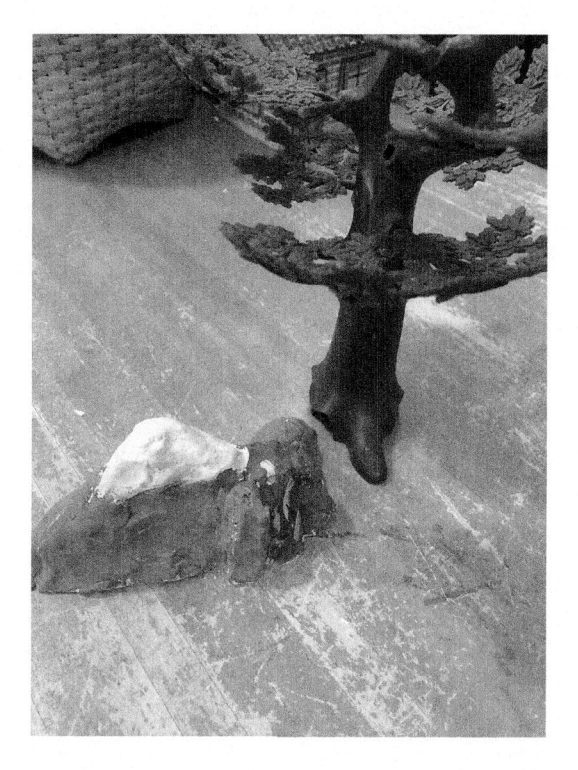

Figure 9.5 Painted clay landscape.

process. The improvised choreography between figures made by the child, or by the child and the therapist together, tells a story. It is as if children sense that they can change and add to their clay, expanding or changing their story as it unfolds. Hass-Cohen and Findley (2015) suggest that: "when experience with the clay is increased, the fear center response is altered into joy" (p. 215). When children create with clay, the strong sensory properties of the material can evoke movement as well as imagery, and children may become very animated. At other times they become calmer and seem more organized as they focus on their clay. Such a sense of calm engenders a greater willingness to carefully save, and then paint, their clay pieces.

I sometimes encourage children's play with clay by working with clay alongside them. Our sharing and watchful "listening" deepens our relationship. One young girl spontaneously created relationships between her clay figures; and she was interested in the simple people or animals that I made in response to her creations. A recurring theme of her art making was friendship and connection, and she explored how relationships can unfold between people or animals who are different, as well as people or animals who are the same. She first created "sisters" in clay, one of whom, "throws up when she is upset." When she played with her figures, we explored emotions and stressors; and thought about ways to moderate stress and feel comfortable. She was able to imagine and create a safe place for her little people, and this also helped her to feel safe. For this child, creating and playing with her creations became a powerful way of articulating her challenges so that she felt supported and could learn coping strategies. When she created animals who were different, she was careful to think about the points of connection between them: what they liked to eat, and what they liked to play. Through sharing art, we share ourselves; and as we looked together at her people and animals, following their interactions with one another, I was able to know her more fully. We worked on ways to increase comfort and connection by building on her strengths as she made new relationships in a new school.

When we create simple forms together, children can connect feeling with their creation. Using clay together allows for a different kind of expression of affect. Children soon sense that they can change their portrayal quickly, or add to it, and this often makes them more willing to experiment.

One child, who was very focused on cars and trucks in all of his drawings and sandtray play, decided to use clay to portray himself, his mother, and the therapist. He carefully worked on these images over two sessions, painting them before sharing them with his mother. He was proud and happy to share this work. He was also visibly proud to share his ability to be more flexible and try something new. Our sharing and watchful "listening" deepened our relationship, and he continued his willingness to try out new materials. The engaging qualities of materials and the creative process allow different expressive languages to enliven one another, and deepens children's experience. When adults carefully observe this experience, the change and flexibility that are enabled for the child can be supported and encouraged.

Clay, Play, and Nature

I once worked with a seven-year-old who was a close and careful observer. At school he was bright and attentive, but he was not always engaged, nor was he communicative about his needs. In the therapy space, he enjoyed using his keen observation skills and explored drawing, painting, and music. He played every instrument in the room, experimenting and carefully listening to their sounds, and engaging in a musical conversation with the therapist. He painted and drew, watching the changes in the colors he mixed with pleasure. He also gathered together objects from the natural world to look at and build with in the sand: stones, crystals, shells, and coral.

He created many worlds in the sand, sifting the sand to make it "snow" as well as "rain." He moved the sand to reveal the watery blue bottom of the tray and talked about how he loved to swim and to sail. As Shore (2006b) has explained, all of a child's senses are essential to their development. The sand is inviting to many children, who literally plunge into the depths of the sand tray. The kinaesthetic process of shifting sand can help a child to feel calm, engaged, and focused. Such play is both developmental and integrative, and seems often to reflect the state of the child who is playing (De Domenico, 2000). This child became interested in using clay after playing in the sand. As is often the way, the processes of expressive and dynamic play and art making complement and encourage one another.

When children are literally "in touch" with materials from the natural world (Lara and Richardson, 2019), as Courtney (2017) has stated, "the varied sensory experiencing of the natural objects has a profound effect upon them" (p. 107). Natural materials help to connect them with what McNiff (2017) describes as, "the sensory dimensions of artistic expression" (p. x). Clay is "a developmental stage of stone and sand," (Courtney, 2017, p. 118) and a material that is literally unearthed. As this child began to experiment with clay, he used the structure of the natural materials from his play in the sand to help organize the form of his clay work. He proceeded in quite a sophisticated fashion, and also in contrast to how he had played in the sand, where he carefully dusted off his fingers after creating patterns and placing figures. Clay was different, and even more direct and tactile. First he created a series of shapes, experimenting and enjoying the colors and properties of the clay without giving his images a name. Together we rolled balls and pushed shapes, rolling, stamping, and squeezing. He explored what happens when clay is hammered, pressed, and curved into shape, without stopping to clean off fingers or hands. His "grammar" of clay included snakes, balls, and squiggles. Such experimental forms embody a child's exploration and energy, as they are explored, recombined, and developed. Working with the "language" of clay, children's "tangible expression through eyes, ears and hands" is "capable of simultaneously constructing and feeling emotion" (Vecchi, 2010, p. 12).

Once he was more experienced, he created a very detailed clay image of his hand.

First, he flattened the clay, adding just enough water. Then, he pressed his hand into the clay, liking, he said, the feeling of the material. He carefully cut around this shape, and smoothed out the edges. Finally, he added another ball of clay at the wrist, articulating the fingers and the way the hand goes into the wrist and the arm. As he worked, he looked back at the natural shapes of a large scallop shell and of a branch coral, both of which connected and then spread gracefully, as the fingers spread out from the hand, and the hand from the wrist. He practiced the careful observation of the scientist or the artist, on a scale and in a way that helped him make sense of the world and his experiences.

Vecchi (2010) has discussed the parallels of children's exploration in the world and with materials with the work of artists, observing how:

> In actual fact, what we define as art is in certain respects closely attuned to children's ways of being: the way they look at the world with great intensity, their greediness to understand it and *inhabit it*. Children and artists, though for different reasons, have the same *completely new way* of seeing when they observe the world.
>
> (p. 114)

This child carefully and thoughtfully experimented with clay. He looked carefully at the natural materials he had used in the sand tray: their shapes, colors, and relations to one another.

Then he created a series of images about which he could tell a story. He built on his observations, in the way of an artist or scientist, and used this basic understanding of materials and processes to support his ability to tell stories through the clay. He built a world in the sand for a cat chosen from the shelves of figures. Then he added a vet, who could take care of animals, standing together with the cat, "who loves the rain." He rained sand down on the cat as he introduced me to his world.

The visual language of clay, the dynamic language of play, and the verbal language of his narrative were interwoven with one another, becoming increasingly complex and expressive. Such connection to feeling is what motivates children to use language, whether verbal or nonverbal, in a meaningful, communicative, fashion. The images created in clay formed the vocabulary of an expressive "language" for this child. Such a language can be used to explore relationships and affect.

The first clay figures he arranged together in relationship to one another were a little ghost and an even smaller cat, which he perched on the ghost's shoulder. He modeled each with great delicacy and care because of their scale. These, he said, were "Scary and Kitty." They were friends, and therefore not frightening to one another. He had played with a friendly ghost and with cats in the sand. With clay, he could depict a different relationship, balancing the two figures together. As this child became more articulate with his use of clay, he was becoming more comfortable in his school environment. He was settling in, even as his little clay beings were settled in to their shared environment. His parents reported that he had new friends at school and was sharing more about his day. Using the language of clay, his stories revealed how his images made possible "a process of empathy relating the self to things and things to each other" (Vecchi, 2010, p. 5).

His clay cats had other adventures. One day, we sat in the sun and made tiny clay eggs to put into an intricate nest. He then created a bird. He arranged his figures carefully to protect the eggs in a nest that was big enough for the cat as well. His cat had a very expressive tail, and he moved it gently onto the edge of the nest full of eggs, looking down without disturbing anything. The cat meowed, still giving the space of the nest to the bird and her eggs, which were never disturbed as the cat came for a visit. "He's a friendly cat," the child explained. He then went to get the big yellow ball stored behind my sofa, to be the sun shining down on the nest. The sun went down, hidden again, as he took out a silk scarf with stars and moon, and lifted a little metal moon into the sky. Eggs and nest, bird and cat, were peacefully at rest.

Chapter 10
From Perfectionism to Playfulness

For autistic children or adolescents with tendencies toward perfectionism, having a way to approach situations that feel ambiguous, and therefore uncomfortable, is essential to establishing a sense of safety. Otherwise, discomfort can arise even in the midst of play or art making that they have been enjoying. They may stop drawing and want to throw their work away. Or they may stop playing, feeling "stuck." They may feel reluctant to accept help, either from the therapist or to metaphorically find "helpers" in their play or to create them in their art.

One young adolescent explained how at school, he sometimes feels he is being treated "like a little kid," but is still expected to behave as an older kid and be responsible. While therapy is a safe environment, and more comfortable than school for many children, this tension between wanting to play "like a little kid" and wanting to feel more mature persists. Older children may say, "I don't know what should happen next" when they are feeling stuck, even in play they have chosen. Younger ones just stop the process entirely. Therapists need to offer support through this confusion and ambiguity so that children's stories can unfold and be appreciated.

One child playing in the doll's house was ready to abruptly stop playing when he could not find one of the myriad of tiny things his children needed. There was an array of food, toys, and other belongings to choose from for the doll house people, as well as materials to create more. With the therapist's encouragement, he was able to find a "helper," Santa Claus, to help bring what was needed to the children, and also to care about the children. This Santa brought presents to the house and also to the children's school, which the child quickly created in another little house "right next door." The children, he said, liked being so close to home when they were in school. For the first time, this child had connected the worlds of home and school through his play. Another child moved his beloved wrestlers into the doll's house, and they expertly took part in gently caring for "baby boys." This nurturing play allowed him, together with the action figures, to explore a new role less focused on competition and winning and more focused on connection and caring. He visibly relaxed as he tucked the babies in with blankets he had decorated for them.

DOI: 10.4324/9781315173306-10

Children and adolescents with autism often need a more robust sense of hope that things which have been hard for them can feel easier. When they report having a "bad day," this may mean that one thing has been especially difficult. Forming more accurate perceptions of their expectations for themselves is essential to instilling a sense of hope.

They need support to understand that their behavior, which is monitored so closely at many schools, consists of what they do, but is also connected to what they are feeling and how they are thinking. When behavior is accepted as a means of communication, that behavior often improves. One child who was inclined to see his days as "all bad" felt more comfortable when he was increasingly able to see the perspectives of others who in turn were more accepting of his perspective. Both his grades and his teacher's comments about positive behaviors increased, and he felt less need for control.

Play is an important way for children to explore greater flexibility and more connection with others. But venturing into play can be difficult for perfectionistic children. An autistic third grader talked about what it is like to play with his peers, and he explained that he does not choose to play with others "who don't know the rules." When we played together, we worked on greater tolerance toward my ignorance of his rules. We explored whether his patience with my learning curve around the rules for baseball could extend to a bit more tolerance of his peers on the playground. He was initially very skeptical about this idea, and also very annoyed with me when I didn't follow the right protocol for the games unfolding on a miniature scale in the sand. We explored new ways to play that would feel comfortable to him. I asked if it would be okay if he taught me the right way, and then I practiced, and he coached.

In an early game he told me: "If I were the head of baseball I would fire you as a ref!" And yet he wanted to play. We connected in play despite my ignorance. He eventually realized that an enjoyable part of being an "expert" himself was teaching me the rules. Over time, he was able to modify the action figures he loved to play with, making them clothes, or adding on details with fabric or clay, rather than rejecting them because they were not exactly "right." Once we had shared active, rule laden, and sometimes aggressive and "scary" play, he was able to focus on coping and calming strategies. He willingly explored a wider range of interactions and emotions through his play. His play in the sand included a "feelings" baseball game. With some prompting and modeling, he gave them expert "coaching" to help with self-regulation. He instructed his team to not be scared, to "calm down," and also not be so angry when they didn't hit a home run. He reminded his team that this would be a good way to focus on their goals. And, at last, he told his team that they would have fun playing, whether they won or lost.

Sometimes art making can help a child to feel more comfortable and better able to tolerate a greater range of affect and ways of understanding their experiences. Sometimes children have a special, preferred way of approaching either the art materials or the process of art making that helps them to move forward and become more flexible. One child chose to sit and trace the outlines of dinosaur figures. Knowing that he had their shape "right" made him feel freer to relax, and then he could carefully and calmly add all the details he was so good at observing. When he tried to draw the dinosaurs without following this sequence, he was visibly tense and worried, and started to become angry. By beginning in this individual way, he was able to move on to more spontaneous drawing.

The calming potential of manipulating materials or creating an image also allows children to articulate what feels scary to them. One young boy presented me with a bad dream, very tentatively. He said, "it's hard to talk about . . . it's too scary." Once we had accomplished the transition of a scary dream onto paper, and then into a portfolio, we were ready to move on to other things. When this young dreamer first came to see me, he was very unhappy at school, and having trouble both with the demands of his program and with making friends. He was increasingly frustrated by the demands of his own perfectionism as well. His insistence on perfect timing, together with an obsession with the passage of time, were also challenges to his parents and teachers. Helping him to become engaged with art was a challenge. He was an observant and graphically adept child, and also very, very knowledgeable about dinosaurs. He was especially desirous that his artwork realize his well-informed high standards, and initially resistant to drawing at all. He would draw a dinosaur and then turn to ask me, "How perfect is this?" Grandin (in Richardson, 2009) has identified how "some kids won't use a talent area because they can't get it absolutely perfect" (p. 111). I was grateful that he was willing to draw. I was also mindful that his initially inflexible approach to creating, focused as he was on the art product being "perfect," could easily undermine the therapy goal of building communication. I wanted to find solutions to challenges, not create challenges. A decrease in perfectionism allows for the regulating "flow" of engaging with materials and communicating through the emerging image.

For perfectionistic children or adolescents, it is helpful to experiment with ways to relax even before making art or choosing what to play. For one child, playing with the bop bag or relaxing on cozy pillows helped him to feel ready to play. He was also able, after moving and relaxing, to talk more about his feelings and to connect through play. He chose puppets who sometimes talked about how they were feeling. The puppets wanted "to be good at things," just like him. Over time, they developed more and more patience with one other. This was paralleled by his tolerance of his therapist's inevitable "mistakes" in our shared puppet play that he loved to direct.

Perfectionistic children and adolescents are usually willing to experiment with relaxation if it is introduced by the therapist at the right moment. Relaxation practice worked particularly well for one child once he had learned some simple techniques and then had a chance to be the "expert." He invited his parents into the office, guiding them through a short relaxation story and reminding them gently to "breathe, Mommy and Daddy." Another child picked up

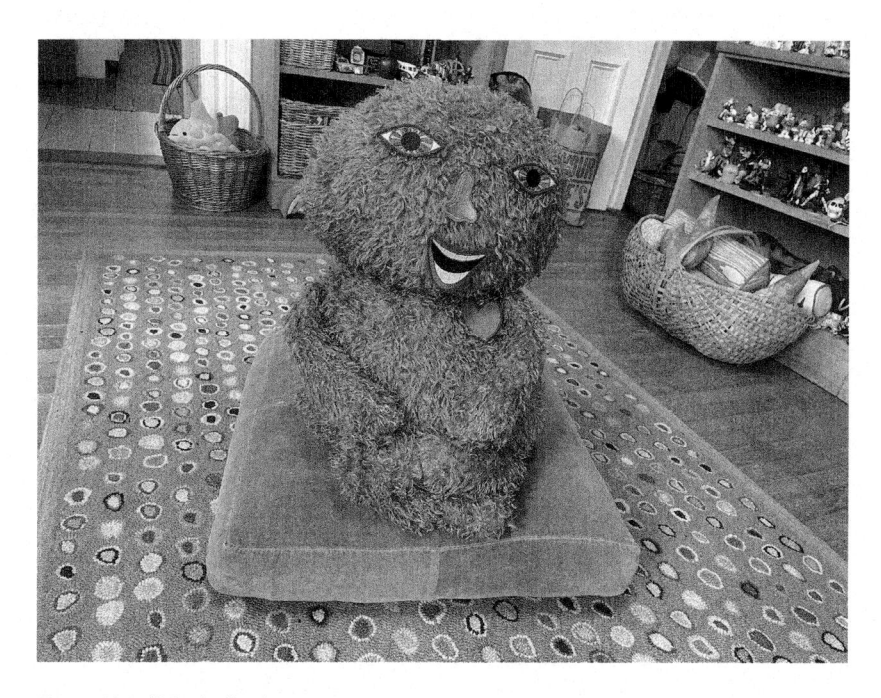

Figure 10.1 "Meebie" relaxes in a yoga pose.

my large purple Meebie figure, arranged him comfortably on the floor, and declared, "now Meebie will do some yoga." Then he settled himself on a cushion alongside Meebie.

As Goldberg (2013) explains, "Emotional upsets trigger the nervous system to activate motor neurons, increasing muscle tension, a habitual pattern for many children with special needs" (p. 63). Children and adolescents with autism may be especially susceptible to stress because of differences in their autonomic nervous systems (Goldberg, 2013), giving rise to self- soothing calming behaviors. Movement, yoga, and relaxation can help them to focus and self- regulate as well as calm down. A wider range of art making and play is then possible.

Drawing and playing together bring the child or adolescent and the therapist into the flow of developing relationship and exploring affect; sometimes drawing together, side by side, or even on the same paper. I was invited by one child to help create a superhero. I followed his lead, carefully drawing at the same speed, and with the same pressure on my crayon that he intently applied on his. Slowly we were able to talk about what happens when even a superhero becomes angry and frustrated. Our superhero, of course, was not the only one dealing with these struggles.

Different materials give children a new kind of freedom to change anything they might not initially approve of. For one child, it was polychrome clay that helped him feel freer to experiment and still maintain his careful sense of detail. Searching for accurate color, he carefully added layers of precisely observed details to the action figures he constructed. Despite some initial hesitation, the kinaesthetic experience of using clay can be very satisfying for perfectionistic children, as they became less fixated on the precision of their imagery, and more engaged in the sensory process of creating. Finding a comfortable fit between their sensory preferences, the image they imagine, and the material itself, allows children to approach making art in a freer and more flexible way. Their pleasure and satisfaction in the process, and satisfaction with what they create, can thus begin to overtake the distress caused by perfectionism.

For a child who delighted in inventing new things from board games to shadow boxes to instruments, I knew that I always needed to have plenty of open-ended materials available. Any given material might be transformed into something else. The sense of our solving a problem together, which delighted him, helped us to build our relationship. I was able to point out how inventive and imaginative he was being. And as he became increasingly willing to work with a challenge in making art, he moved further away from perfectionism, to create with less frustration and a greater sense of engagement and fun. He loved being the expert, the one with all the good ideas, and he could accept some imperfections as long as we both tried hard to get things right. We worked on the right color, the right gesture, and the right relationship of figures in space. In this, he was a true artist.

He had not been interested in play in the sand tray, although it intrigued him as a potential hiding place for small toys. This response to the sensory properties of materials is individual, and it is essential to observe the child's response and to accommodate. Grandin (in Attwood, 2000) described how the process of "dribbling sand through my hands" was calming to the extent that she could engage her senses to feel regulated before connecting with the outside world again. She described to Tony Attwood (2000) how she would "watch the sand, studying each little particle like a scientist looking at it under a microscope. When I did that I could tune the whole world out." She added, "you know, I think it's OK for an autistic kid to do a little bit of that, because it's calming."

The sand does not have a similar calming effect on all children, and this particular child did not wish to touch the sand at all. And yet, he needed, as everyone needs in therapy, "a place where they can feel safe," as Cohen has described (Cohen et al., 1995, p. 106). Natural materials sometimes serve as a comforting counterbalance to perfectionistic tendencies: they are perfect, just as they are, and they engage the senses. In a study contrasting natural materials with art materials, Chang and Netzer described how children felt more "spontaneous, imaginative, creative, and relaxed" (in Swank et al., 2020, p. 157) when creating with natural materials. This child enjoyed exploring the baskets of natural materials in the room and painting on rocks. I suggested he put one of the paper boats we had been folding in an empty tray, with its blue bottom that looked like water. True to form, he wanted to actually fill the tray with water, which we did, rather than "pretending" that the blue base was the water. He chose toys from the shelf of sand tray images to add to the tray—the first time he had done this—and added a small rowboat, and then a child, traveling through the watery landscape. He looked at me with a smile, as if he was taking note of my response to this unprecedented play which included a young boy, like him.

Some children move, not from play to art, but from art to play. This child, for the first time, was able to play in the "world" he had created, adding a lighthouse, sea creatures, rocks, and another boat, together with the boy who, he reminded me, was "not real." As Wolfberg (2003) suggests, pretend play is learned by autistic children, and often experienced through the support and presence of another who is ready to join in the play. While this child reminded me that the person in his sand tray was not real, and could not talk, he still enjoyed creating this world, and the action and the story within it. He allowed me to share in his play, both witnessing his activity and providing supports and materials. We kept a delicate balance of engaging with one another and respecting the "rules" of the play, even while we moved toward more flexibility.

Sometimes older children question the role of play in their therapy altogether. While they are often drawn to the art materials, toys, and puppets, and may especially enjoy the array of "fidgets" that feel good to touch, or absorbing to look at after a long day at school, they seem to be asking, and sometimes literally do ask, "is it okay to play?" Willingness to play with fidgets can lead into more expressive and interactive play. When children play with expanding sphere balls, for example, they both enjoy their rhythm, and use them to calm down. Sometimes children will practice breathing with the ball, and older children like seeing these tools as "strategies" for calming, a word that feels more adult. This sensory engagement helps with acknowledging worries or concerns.

Older children feel the need for balance between their need to play, to use sensory comforts, or to express themselves through puppets or sandtray figures or art, and their very appropriate desire to be treated as an older kid who is more mature. For one child who was working on ways to cope with worries and anxiety, talking through difficult moments with an adult was sometimes helpful, both at home and school. He was so diligent about addressing his challenges that he wondered if it was really okay for him to be more relaxed, and to play or draw in a session as well as talk. Envisioning a "worry meter" as a visual representation of how worries accumulate and accelerate was a helpful bridge between talking, art making, and playing. He felt respected in his effort to understand and take greater control of stressors.

One of the requirements for a collection of images for Sandtray/Worldplay is that the choice of images should provide enough psychological depth for an adult to play in the sand in a meaningful way. In fact, parents sometimes use

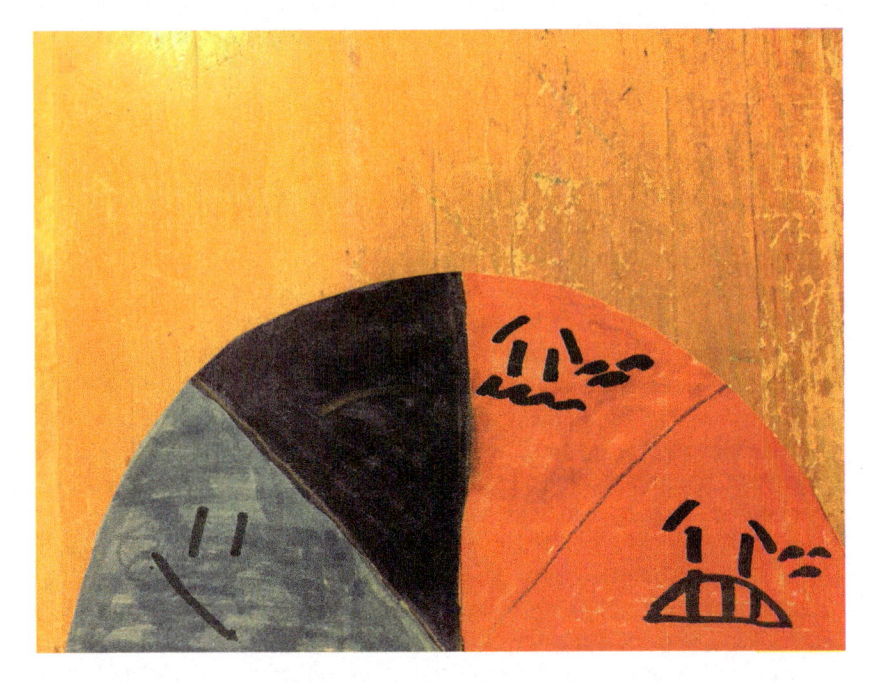

Figure 10.2 The worry meter.

the sand tray, as do teens and young adults. Knowing that people older than they are also playing helps to give children permission for this process.

A young adolescent who enjoyed looking at the sandtray images in his first session was happy to find cartoon figures that he liked, but he did not want to play with them. He told me, "I'm a really good artist," taking out the sketchbook he was carrying with him, which had a picture of one of the characters on my shelves. He was indeed adept at drawing and he also knew everything about the history of Mickey Mouse. While he drew, he communicated very directly about the things he liked to do, and began to touch on the things that were hard to do.

Another child used my monkey puppet very expressively, with evident enjoyment. However, he felt that if I used a puppet to respond to him it would be too "babyish," and therefore not comfortable for him. Through this play we both came to understand what was comfortable, not only for the monkey, but also for the child himself. He made the monkey try out, and then reject, places to be in the room, different things to "eat," different activities to engage in, and who he wanted to be with. Such reflection helps children to make a wider range of choices in the therapy setting, choices that can allow them to address their challenges. Creating comfort with the idea of play and movement in the therapy room is important for any child who "wants not to worry" so much. When tentative children decide, as one child did, after first drawing and then talking about his drawing, "now I want to play, I think that will help me," there can be movement in therapy as well as in the child's body as they move more freely through the environment.

After many sessions, another child decided he was ready to explore the sand tray. He quickly created what it would be like to be "sinking in quicksand." He explored ways out of the quicksand. Once he had begun to play, he was very animated and communicative with me. He liked the notion that sometimes we get ideas for our lives from our play in the sand tray. These new ideas can help us to create change or comfort.

When autistic children or adolescents can play freely without being fearful that this is not appropriate, themes of exploration and mastery tend to appear in their play. As they master fears and try new things in play, carefully setting up environments to be explored, there is a parallel decrease in fearfulness and anxiety. They are able to regulate affect and shift their focus through their play. Often, children report less depressed affect and lessened anxiety once they have relaxed into the process of play. Children gain insights that help them to relax their expectations of themselves and feel more open to change. The same is true of making art.

One very peaceful day, a child looked up from an elaborate crayon drawing to say, "some people . . . have a hard time drawing because they rush too much . . . if they're not a good drawer." He explained, "I don't rush . . . my teacher knows which one is mine even without my name . . . because I go slow." He then stood up to demonstrate what he meant. He began jumping up and down, loudly saying, "no no no, it's not good!" He grimaced and asked me, "does anyone do that here?" He shared his advice about how to help other children "slow down." "You can," he encouraged me, "tell them, calm down, or say, you could do it over again . . . one thing you could do, is they could go slow around the edges." Here he demonstrated how he carefully moves color across the outer surface of a drawing and deliberately makes his color choices. The responsive quality of his outline, and thoughtful addition of colors was striking, as he worked carefully but in a relaxed fashion. Then he recalled my suggestion about "really really looking" at what you want to draw, and added, "what else I do, is, I try to see it in my head." He said that drawing is something he really likes to do; perhaps not as much as computer games—"I live for that!"—but both drawing and "making things," he declared, definitely belong on the short list of things he likes the most.

He used his artwork and creative inventions to address our relationship to one another. One day, he became very angry at me, and was literally in my face and yelling, "You wanted me to miss science! I didn't get to do an experiment! You made the appointment at the wrong time!" At his next appointment, he came in with a present for me. This was a noisemaker, a shaker with a picture of a gorilla, with crumpled paper and other objects inside. It made a low rumble when I shook it. His construction was labeled "gorilla noise." In fact, it made far less noise than he did himself when he became angry. We talked about the "rumbling" stage of feeling angry. Together we wondered how it could help to know when we were rumbling, and to seek help with uncomfortable feelings before they grew too hard to handle. We played with his shaker together. I experimented with adding in some louder drums. He concluded that maybe, since we did like to be together that I was trying to help him with his own "rumbling." And then he suggested that perhaps I had not made him miss a favorite activity intentionally. Toward the end of therapy, he reflected on the time we had spent together making art. He declared, "you could be the best inventor . . . we're like a team . . . two inventors . . . we could make things and help people." Then he added, "you made the best boats . . . but I have the good ideas!" What a wonderful image of our work together, and of our relationship, this blending of art, play, and wonderful ideas.

Chapter 11

Empathy

Understanding the Other Through Art and Play

Empathy is essential to understanding the perspective of another person, on both an affective and a cognitive level. Empathy is a dynamic, relational process, which involves going beyond understanding what another person is thinking to engaging through the body and emotions, as well as the mind. When this complex process of understanding the thoughts and feelings of another person engages children and adolescents with autism, they can be acutely sensitive and also empathic. They can then use their senses to better understand the meaning of what they are feeling themselves. Barron-Cohen and Wheelwright (2004) explain that for people with autism, as for anyone:

> Empathy is without question an important ability. It allows us to tune in to how someone else is feeling or what they might be thinking. Empathy allows us to understand the intentions of others, predict their behavior, and experience emotion triggered by their emotion. In short, empathy allows us to interact effectively in the social world. It is also the "glue" of the social world, drawing us to help others and stopping us from hurting others.
>
> (p. 163)

Emotional regulation and enhanced communication are important goals in therapy with autistic children and adolescents. Regulation supports the level of comfort needed for empathic thoughts, feelings, and behaviors. Nader-Grosbois and Mazzone (2014) found that when children with autism are able to regulate their emotions and communicate better, that they are also more able to take the perspective of others; a perspective that supports the growth of empathy.

I have had children with autism notice my face while they are telling me a story, and wonder if what they had told me might be making me feel sad, or whether I am just thinking about what they have said. And children are similarly curious about other children they might see coming to or leaving a therapy session, asking questions like, "what does that girl come here for?" One child suggested that another child entering the waiting room as they were

DOI: 10.4324/9781315173306-11

leaving might be worried, just like them. Children are visibly comforted by this assurance that many children have worries and sad feelings, and that they also come to get help with those feelings. They seem to feel less alone with their challenges, and to sense that the materials and processes of play and art making will help them to resolve these challenges. As Vygotsky (in Penfold, 2019) has described:

> the more a child sees, hears, and experiences, the more he knows and assimilates, the more elements of reality he will have in his experience, and the more productive will be the operation of his imagination.
>
> (p. 15)

The sensory and expressive potential of play and art making are rich sources for communication and the growth of empathic understanding.

The kinaesthetic and sensory aspects of making art can help children to move through challenging feelings and behaviors and build connection and communication. On a day when a child did not want to play or make art in my therapy room, we went outside to tell our stories with chalk, where we were freer to move around. While initially complaining that this activity was boring, he soon became interested in tracing hands, feet, and even bodies. He responded increasingly to me, and became interested in how he was portraying himself with the traced outline of his body, and he agreed to both draw inside his own outline and share some things about himself. His affect brightened, and his engagement increased, and he became more interested in telling his story, and responding to the drawing I was making alongside him.

A young adolescent described to me how he used empathic understanding to comfort his younger sister, first sensing that she was upset, and then thinking about what he could do to help her feel better. He both responded to how she was feeling on an affective level, and thought carefully about why she might be feeling sad, and what he could do to help. His support was a mix of affective and sensory comfort, as he sat with her and patted her on her back. He also gave her support on a cognitive level, telling her jokes to distract her and make her laugh and feel better after sharing her laughter. This boy felt calm enough to respond to the needs of his sister and to understand her perspective. Her appreciation of his presence, in turn, encouraged his empathic response.

The behavior of others shapes subsequent behavior, and the construction of empathic relationships is a mutual process that needs to be supported within the family and the community as well as in therapy. Stern (1985) discusses the process of creating "a shared framework of meaning" (p. 136) as foundational to all children's development. Children and adolescents with autism need support not only for their own growing empathic awareness, but also because, while it may be difficult for them to "mind read" the thoughts and intentions of others, the minds of autistic children and adolescents are difficult for others to "read" as well. This creates the "double empathy problem" described by

Milton (2012), wherein the lack of full understanding of the other, and subsequent lapse of communication, are not solely limited to the autistic individual. The phenomenon of the double empathy problem suggests that neurotypical people and autistic people have difficulty understanding one another on both sides, because their perceptions and experiences are very different. In responding to people with autism, there is, then, "a dynamic interaction between the individual and how others perceive and react to that individual" as Jaswal and Akhtar (2018, p. 2) have explained.

Empathy is a relational and transactional process. Mitchell (2016) notes that the behavior of others always shapes how an individual behaves, whether they are autistic or not. But as Jaswal and Akhtar (2018) have observed:

> altered interactions may deprive autistic children of the kinds of experiences thought to be necessary for typical language and social development, and they may deprive autistic children and adults of opportunities to develop strong social relationships which have important mental and physical health benefits.
>
> (p. 2)

and which promote the growth of mutual empathy. Creating what Gallese (2009) terms a "neurally instantiated we-centric space," allows for sharing "actions, intentions, feelings and emotions with others, thus grounding our identification with and connectedness to others" (p. 520). The conditions for empathic understanding must be present in therapy as they are in optimal early relationships.

A bright and observant young boy with a love for and careful attention to all things that go found the location of my office on a major crosstown street a source of great interest. He noticed every siren that went past the window even from the second floor, with windows closed and air conditioning on. Coupled with his sensitivity to sound, such that the subtle sound of my cooling and heating system would always startle him, we worked on establishing his comfort in this new environment. I helped him to notice that the warm or cool air blows UP in the waiting room, and DOWN from the ceiling in my upstairs room in a century old building; and to anticipate how and when this might happen. I wanted to increase his comfort with a change in the sound level and temperature. We went downstairs and watched paper blow up from the floor over the waiting room grate, and went back upstairs to trace where the air travelled. Helping him to feel more in control of the environment helped him feel more comfortable with me. For both typically developing children, and children with autism, greater empathy seems to be possible when they are experiencing fewer sensory processing difficulties and less stress. As Tortora (2006) describes, "How children regulate their emotional reactions and how their emotions are displayed physically can be expressed in how they hold and move their bodies" (p. 460). We worked on establishing comfort in a number of ways, from using familiar and pleasurable art materials to paying attention to what might happen outside of the room itself as we moved through the therapy space. While we couldn't anticipate the arrival of traffic outside, we certainly could anticipate that this would happen while he was in his session. He always wanted to look out my windows when he caught sight of an interesting truck, so we practiced doing this without rushing and knocking over his chair in the process. My goal was to make this unfamiliar situation feel safe and comfortably familiar by supporting him in accessing greater physical comfort as well as acknowledging his thoughts and emotions in the new situation.

His intense focus on his special interests, and his efforts to become comfortable in a sensory world that sometimes threatened to overwhelm him, made addressing his comfort, and helping him to communicate when he needed help, important goals for our work together. When he was feeling particularly uncomfortable, there were angry outbursts and difficult confrontations with others. He decided that he really liked the toys and art materials in my office, so much so that when we ended our first session together, even after a substantial time to transition, he attempted to kick me on his way out the door because his time was coming to an end. Fortunately, I was able to grab a large pillow to hold in front of my legs, and did not get hurt, thus maintaining my rule that "nobody gets hurt" in the office, which is a safe space. I realized that we needed more structure and predictability in our time together. And he seemed to realize that we would keep spending time together, and that he would have a chance to do the things he had enjoyed again. We arranged a picture sequence for our sessions to support him through the transitions from school, to therapy, and back home. We included what was to come, beginning with drawing, painting, or working with clay together, or telling a story: anything, as long as we were engaged together. We left time for play in the sand tray or making music, ending with cleaning up and then meeting his mother. I made it very clear where he had a choice: in what materials to use, and whether he wanted to play or make art. I also made it clear where he did not have a choice: in cleaning up, and in following my one non-negotiable rule, which is, "nobody gets hurt." At the end of his little book we glued in a photograph of his mother taken in the office. In the image he chose, she sat in the sunlight with a proud and welcoming smile, to remind him that she would be happy to see him, and interested in what he had created if he wanted to share.

During our time together, as he repeatedly jumped up from my table to track the path of an ambulance or police car, I repeatedly helped him to feel comfortable and ready to return to his drawing or playing again. We began to wonder together about what might be going on outside the window. Was someone being helped by the ambulance? Where was the fire truck going? What were the helpers doing, and how did they know what to do? Were they, perhaps, keeping people, including us, safe? I joined in his interest in the trucks we watched together. We engaged through his images based on his special interests, working with shared enthusiasm for the interest and the image alike.

Special interests, like this child's fascination with trucks, can serve many functions in the imaginations of children with autism. Attwood (1997) has discussed how special interests can provide calm, consistency, and a sense of mastery as well as being highly engaging for a child. The ability to focus, to an acute and exclusive extent, on a special interest can also, as Lovecky (2006) has observed, help children to feel more creative and engaged. And this greater understanding of objects outside of themselves can be used to support a greater awareness of others and of emotions.

Joint sessions with a parent and child are an opportunity to build flexibility in responding to one another. They can also provide alternative ways of communicating when behavior has been challenging. As Goucher (2012) suggests, "the act of engaging in one's environment through creative means or through use of traditional art media requires an individual to be, even for a moment, in the social world, open to interaction with another" (p. 295). The presence of the parent or the therapist encourages venturing into this social world, moving from the child's base of comfort with preferred materials, experiences, or interests, into sharing these experiences and interests in a reciprocal fashion, and building on them together.

Children's creating, playing, and sharing can be "an offer of interest," in the words of one parent of a preschooler, an opening through which the adults in a child's life can build a deeper sense of connection, engagement, and meaningful communication. Sometimes the initial "offer" from a child is very subtle. At other times, a child might be more clearly inviting a response from an adult, as when a child brought in a photo album of his visit to an airshow to show me. Together we looked at pictures of him sitting in a helicopter and smiling. We talked about the airplanes he had seen, and then I gently steered the conversation to his presence in these pictures, his look of excitement, and his ability to share a special experience with his family. We looked at his mother's face in the pictures, and talked about whether she had been happy to bring her son to this special, long-awaited event and whether she might be proud of him for earning this opportunity for himself through positive behavior. This spontaneous sharing of his photograph album allowed us to work with one of the central techniques of Weiser's (1999) phototherapy, using photographs others have taken of the client as a catalyst to access their inner feelings more accurately. For a very visual autistic child, such literal affirmation of his own and his mother's affect in the context of a shared special experience was powerful and meaningful. The actual image of this experience encouraged deeper communication. He enjoyed sharing photographs that were precious to him, and his stories.

In a family session, he explored his special interest in a way that included his mother, rather than in a narrowly focused way that excluded her. While he filled his sky with carefully detailed airplane after airplane, with no room for any people, his mother also drew an airplane, flying through a lively landscape "to visit with him." They agreed that the airplanes, aside from being exciting in and of themselves, were also important because they could bring people who loved one another together. Slowly, he moved into greater expression and a greater range of affect.

One day, I told this child who loved airplanes and trucks the story of a huge hook and ladder truck that had parked on the sidewalk across the street from my office, and mentioned how I wished he were there that day to see this unusual event. I knew that he would be able to figure out what was going on, and I told him that. Connecting through special interests, and moving toward more reciprocal or shared interests, can begin with receptivity and sharing from the therapist. He appreciated my sharing this story; and he especially appreciated my curiosity about why a firetruck would be there, on the sidewalk. After we conjectured about the firetruck for a few minutes, he asked, "were you worried about me when there was all that thunder?" He had been at camp the previous day during a thunderstorm. I explained that I had thought about him being at camp, and also that I knew his mother would only send him to a camp where they would keep him safe, even in thunder.

We talked about what he had been doing at camp, and then he became curious about what I had been doing. I had just been out of the office for a prolonged time. He said that his mother had told him that my father was sick, so I had to visit him, and help him; and I could not be here to see children the way I usually did. When I am away from the office, I always let children know in advance. He decided that this was very important, because children want to know what they are going to do and where they are going to be. Nevertheless, he seemed to understand that this absence was one I could not anticipate and tell him about before I left. He was able to accept this lapse on my part without anger.

In one of the most moving moments in my life as a therapist, he then asked, "what happened to your father?" I explained that my father was very, very old, and that he had died. Anticipating a possible frightened reaction, I explained that this had not been painful or scary, even though it was sad, and that I had been there to keep my father company. He thought carefully, and then asked, "Is your father in heaven?" If so, he wanted to know how he had gotten up there. Staying with the animated, reciprocal conversation, I asked how HE thought my father might have gotten there. "In a hot air balloon" he said with a big smile. Here he was thinking about someone important to me, as well as of the hot air balloon that was captivating to him. I felt connected to this child, and I could feel his empathic concern. As I told my story of where I had been, and he told me his story about what might have happened to my father, we communicated on an affective as well as the cognitive level of his more complex storytelling. He both seemed to sense that I was feeling something different from my usual state, and also perhaps sensing that while I would tell him the truth, I also didn't want him to feel frightened. We sat together quietly, sharing this moment with appreciation.

These deeply felt shared experiences are not shared solely through language. Kinaesthetic empathy, as Cardillo explains (personal communication, August 12, 2020), goes deep to encompass the therapist's own bodily experience while observing and experiencing being with another person. A fuller sense of being with one another comes through such sensing and internally responding to one another. I sat quietly with this child, and he sat calmly as well. Berger describes this process as "empathic body connection" (in Nemetz, 2006, p. 104). Franklin (2017) has discussed the importance of extending empathy to both what is being created and what is observed through the art making process. These dimensions of empathy go beyond words. Following our conversation about my father, this young boy began to draw bigger and bigger trucks, flatbed tow trucks that help the "hurt cars" following a big accident. He began to consider, and talk about, how these vehicles functioned with each other, and also helped people. He created "lots of room for cars. They can help everyone," but he also pointed out that not all of the cars on the scene of an accident had been "hurt." We explored the story of what was happening in his images. We thought about the physicality of the trucks, about the process of helping, and then we moved to emotions. Staying with his enthusiasm for the images he created, and experiencing them together, helped us to work together on a deeper level.

He soon made the transition to the sand tray to build a world and play within it. This play became, as with his drawing and sharing process, more animated and relational as he moved more freely through the space. As usual, he chose an array of vehicles: firetruck, tow truck, ambulance, and cars, but he also, for the very first time, took out a basket of people to join the world of the trucks. He selected someone to go in the back of the ambulance, and a helper for the injured people. These were the people from the scenes created in his earlier drawings, and he continued to add what they needed to heal into his world in

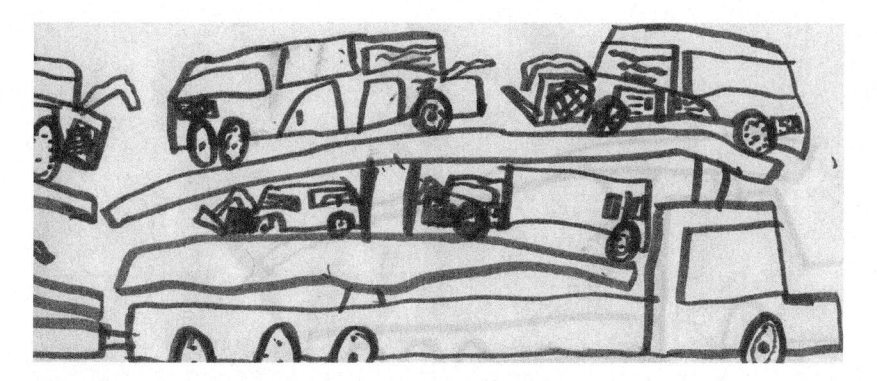

Figure 11.1 A car carrier full of "helping vehicles."

the sand. His exploration of relationships through his art allowed him to experience himself as more connected and caring. After creating the drawings of helping vehicles, he was both more eager, and able, to elaborate on the themes that emerged in the sand, sustaining the empathic communication that had taken place while he was drawing and moving into active engagement.

Chapter 12
Potential and Possibility for Adolescents

An adolescent girl sat in the sun streaming through my office windows. She reflected on a beautiful morning when she awoke early. She described, so vividly that I could visualize this scene myself, the atmosphere of a place in nature where she felt at peace. She focused on the quality of the light and the movement of the breeze—how there was a glow in the sky, and mist rising through the air. When I suggested she try drawing to capture the image, she said, "It's beyond a picture." She was, however, willing to work on capturing the colors. She slowly and thoughtfully chose pastels from a large box to find the color of the atmosphere, and the contrast between the glowing light and the rising mist. To help her get started, I also chose a selection of soft colors based on her description of the scene, mixing them together to try and produce the shimmering light she described. As I made a small drawing alongside her, I demonstrated that it was not necessary to portray the scene literally. I hoped that in capturing the color and feel of a special place, her own image would prove to be calming and self-affirming. She created a tiny drawing with the very "glow" that she had described. Her image was as subtle as the rising mist and impossible to capture in a photograph.

In contrast to the elusive depth of this girl's image, an adolescent boy created a series of strong black and white images of a young man. He began to rip around the edges of the drawings, making the central figure smaller and smaller. This, he said, is how it feels to be teased; as if others are tearing away something from you. Quickly moving to the sand tray, he chose superhero figures. Although they were strong and steady, even superheroes were not immune to teasing in the play that followed. Captain America, he said, had to make a plan for how he could remain steadfast. Even a superhero needs to work to stay strong. Sometimes, he said, a superhero needs to try out a new solution, or to find helpers and friends. We talked about "what superheroes do out in the world." He decided they need to practice to meet challenges, just like he needed to practice to learn new things. And "sometimes," he observed, "then we can do things we didn't think we can!"

Balancing play, art making, and sometimes, talk, is an ongoing process with adolescents navigating the anticipated developmental challenges of

DOI: 10.4324/9781315173306-12

adolescence. Initial sessions can suggest possibilities for communication. Looking at the figures used for play in the sand tray provides a visual introduction to therapy, since there are so many choices that most adolescents will find something that speaks on their level. One boy found a figure of Mickey Mouse at the start of his first session. I discovered that he knew everything about the history of Mickey Mouse, and we created a connection through this character. As we looked together at his drawings of Mickey, carefully observed and rendered, we acknowledged his strengths. Building on strengths provides a base to address challenges. While adolescents may not always articulate their worries, fears, or anxious feelings in initial sessions, sometimes these are expressed very clearly. This young artist expressed a wish to worry less and to feel more comfortable at school. Before we ended, I invited him to take a stone from my collection of white beach rocks and create an image to keep. He created colorful "Mickey faces" and put the rock in his pocket to take home. He told me that he knew about "worry stones," and suggested "maybe I could put some of my worries . . . into Mickey."

The experiences and emotions adolescents depict through art making and play can be intense. One boy described his awareness of this intensity, saying, "I know I will have some of those touch feelings." I wondered what this meant and whether these are feelings that touch you more strongly than others, and he agreed. Exploring emotions, relationships, and boundaries with others can

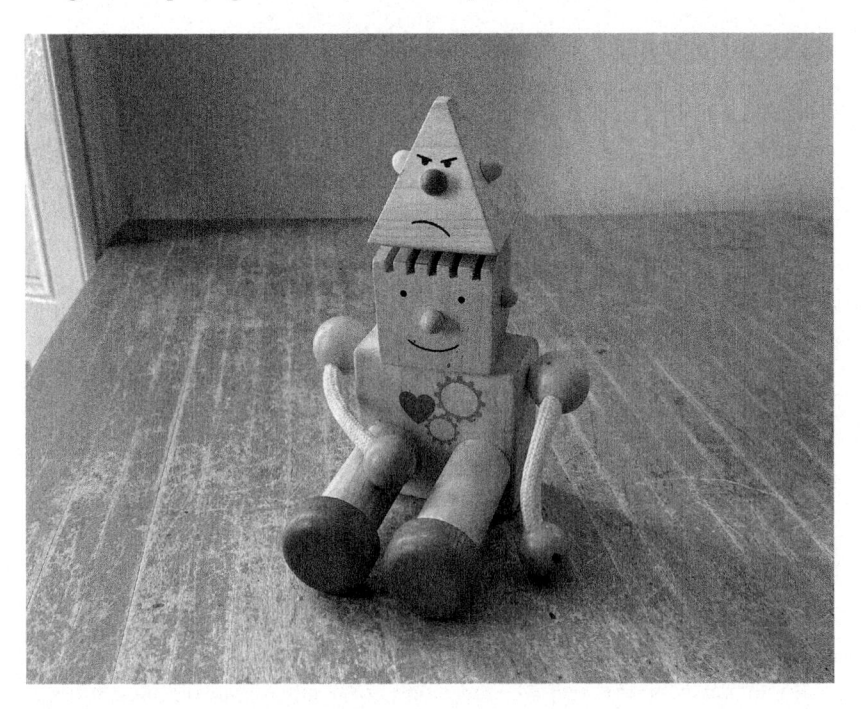

Figure 12.1 Robot with mixed feelings.

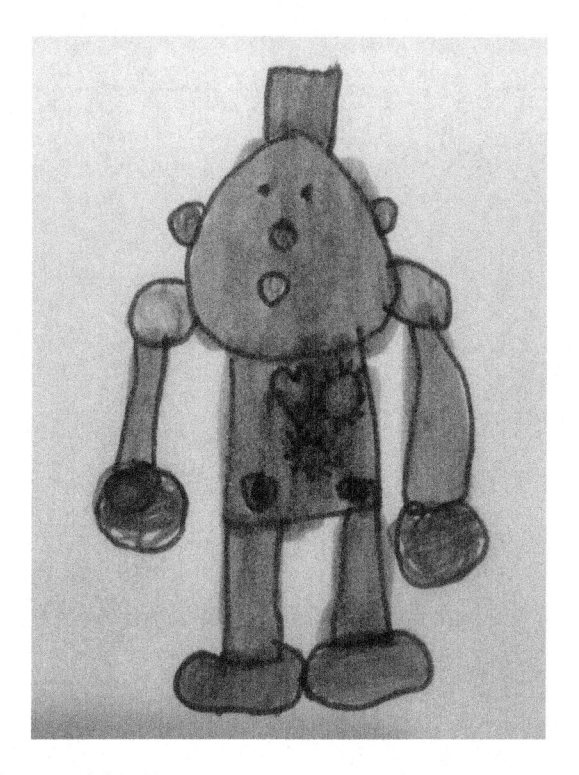

Figure 12.2 Portrait of the robot.

be a difficult process for autistic adolescents. Gotham (in Weinstock, 2019) suggests that, finding "strategies that could effectively redirect people with autism from dwelling on negative information . . . can help them develop a more adaptive pattern of thinking" (p. 1). Mixed emotions can be particularly challenging for any adolescents to understand. Using visual imagery helps with this process through clarifying the different emotional elements involved.

A robot with changeable heads was used by one boy to portray a character he called, "Mr. Good/Bad." Mr. Good/Bad could be unpredictable, the way friends, and even teachers, could be unpredictable and confusing. His own characters in his drawings or in his sandtray play showed very clear emotions, announcing: "It happens that I'm angry right now!" As his figures moved through the sand he said, "that's the sound they make when they're angry." And another character explained "I can only feel happy, I don't have any other emotion." But the unpredictable and changeable Mr. Good/Bad was more difficult to understand. After playing, he created a series of trading cards. He decided that these characters were "mixed up" and not easy to read at first glance.

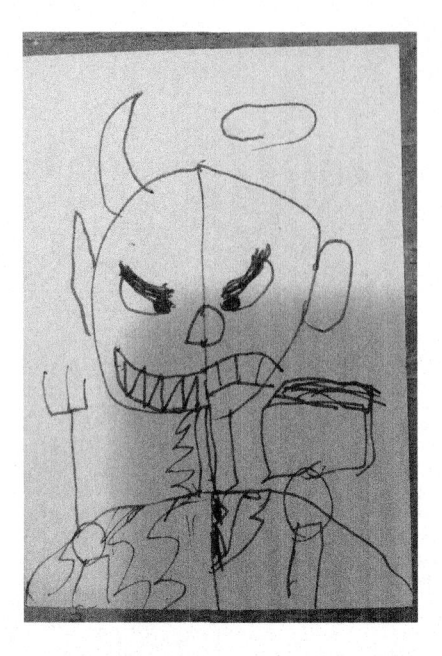

128 Potential and Possibility for Adolescents

Figure 12.3 Mixed feelings: scared and angry.

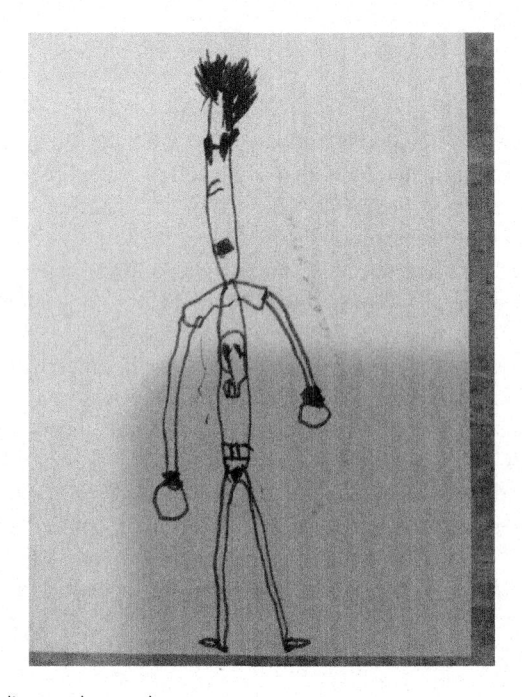

Figure 12.4 Trading card: a cool teen.

"It's mixed up," he explained, because "a good smile can be a bad smile." Since Mr. Good/Bad did not talk, careful observation was the only way to understand what he really meant, even when he didn't immediately "make sense." His creation of a three-dimensional figure incorporating all the mixed feelings had helped him to make more sense of a confusing situation that he explored further through drawing.

After talking about his images, we took time to relax after this hard work. He agreed that I could read a relaxing story (Khalsa, 1998) and he chose one set on the beach. He listened thoughtfully as he let the sand from the sand tray run through his fingers, imagining a seagull coming to eat from his hand. Then he took out my rain stick and we listened together to the soft, rhythmical sound. He announced, "Now I feel better."

Directing attention into the body helps adolescents to identify what an emotion feels like and where this feeling is in their body. Relaxation and reflection support self-awareness through helping adolescents to feel a connection between their body and their brain. The goal is to help the adolescent to feel more centered and more comfortable. For adolescents with neurological challenges, there is a tendency to habitually function under stress. Emotions and physical sensations are both involved in this process, and may be manifested in drawings or through play. Sometimes adolescents need encouragement to process stressors on this bodily level. When there is tension or distress remaining after creating an image, relaxation can provide closure to a session, teaching skills that can be used for calming and managing stress. While relaxation is introduced by the therapist, it is essential to tune in to both the adolescent's need for regulation and calming and their readiness to begin. Khalsa (2016) has noted the importance of "seeing what moves them"—what they are interested in, and then using "creativity to introduce an activity that is similar" (p. 122). One boy's personal and creative response to the invitation to relax was to connect with the peaceful rhythm of the sand running through his hands and the sound of the rain stick.

Relaxation can also be supported through the choice of materials for a session. Adolescents often choose their art materials with particular care, searching for precisely the right width and weight of black line, or the right balance between flow and control of color as it moves across the page. "Imagine," suggests Davis (2017) "a nervous teenager drawn to colored pencils forming scratchy lines" (p. 66) as they create a drawing from nature. Through staying with the process, they can connect to a place, an image, and themselves, as the scratchiness of the initial drawing becomes smoother and more fluid. Sometimes drawings vary so widely in their pressure and intensity so as to appear as if created with entirely different materials. The process of drawing can become so intense that the paper itself is destroyed as more and more colors and strokes are added.

Intently drawing may first reflect, and then help to let go of tension. Anxiety and depression are common symptoms for adolescents with autism (Bromfield,

2010; Attwood, 2006; Richardson, 2009). It is a clinical challenge to create a sense of movement and self- efficacy for them. Anxiety or depressed mood readily manifests in worries, fears, or fixations, whether these fixations are focused on a particular event or are experienced as a persistent repetitive state. Recent studies have found that, "repetitive thinking about negative events and emotions can also set some autistic people up for a depressive episode" (Weinstock, 2019, p. 1). Focused interests can be comforting, as can repetitive behaviors, but focusing repeatedly on negative events is distressing. Experiencing a sense of movement and possibility in therapy can help young people with autism, as Bromfield (2010) suggests, "in ways that go beyond alleviating the specific symptom," (p. 180) by suggesting an alternative view of the self. This alternative and broader view of the self also helps to counter the developmental challenges of intimacy and isolation. As Elkis-Abuhoff (2009) has observed, these challenges are amplified for adolescents with autism, and may be manifested in their imagery or stories. Opening up communication and reducing stress through art and play helps adolescents cope with developmental challenges, including the communication and sensory challenges of autism, through discovering and using their strengths.

Exploring materials parallels exploring the emotional content of imagery. "I think I need paint for this," one girl declared, as she was experimenting with pastels on paper. Her use of pastels followed a series of initial doodles made with a new range of markers that she enjoyed, but ultimately rejected, as "all wrong" for the feeling she wanted to create. She carefully chose a wide brush and began to layer gouache with broad sweeps across her paper. Making swirling strokes, she allowed the colors to mix. Beginning with a layer of blue, she commented, "I need a bigger space . . . and I need more than just blue." She began to add rose and purple to her painting, at first soft and watery, and then more vibrant. With a strong stroke, she added a vivid contrast of red orange paint. "There is anger," she observed. She added more water and allowed the color to move and change, diluting the feeling of anger together with the paint. "I'm not sure how I did that!" she exclaimed, as she watched the changing colors. The freedom to move beyond the expectation of perfection is built in to water-based media, whose flow will continue, whether it is wanted or not. She experimented with taking color out and adding it in again, very deliberately. Standing back from her finished painting she observed how the colors had mixed and transformed. I suggested that perhaps they mixed the way she had described her feelings mixing as she continued the process of painting and reflection.

Adolescent clients have sometimes described painting as calming and absorbing, akin to a "flow state" (Csikszentmihalyi, 2008), where they are absorbed and engaged in both the moment and in the process. Kapitan (2013) observed a similar process in adolescents with autism, observing how art therapy provided "a relaxed yet focused experience," that she suggests exemplifies "art therapy's sweet spot between art, anxiety, and the flow experience"

(p. 54). The willingness to loosen the grip on a pencil, or loosen the control over an image, allows for the creation of an image that, in the words of one young painter, can be "slowly released" after first visualizing it "in your head" (Richardson, 2009, p. 103). Such transformation through the art making process, as Chilton and Wilkinson (2017) suggest, "channels anxiety, transforms chaotic energy, and promotes concentration" (p. 103).

I sometimes join in the process of drawing or painting, setting a precedent of working more freely, suggesting, and also demonstrating, that it's okay to not be perfect. Sometimes adolescents have a strong preference for very controlled media, together with high expectations for how their finished image should look. On a day that we had been talking about confusing feelings, an intent adolescent girl watched me layer blue and violet on a small sheet of paper, cover them with black in some places, and introduce a little red. I asked her, "if the colors were feelings, any feelings," could she tell where those feelings were starting to change? "That's starting to look a little mad," she exclaimed, as the red became stronger. "I can see where it's starting." We then talked about the relatively calm sweeps of blue and violet, some of her favorite colors, and what happened when the other colors began to mix and change within the space of the drawing. She decided my drawing looked "quieter." Keeping our focus on the drawing together was a way of creating comfort. She then was able to draw herself, visibly enjoying the release of pressure to create something perfect.

Another girl explained her rainbow lexicon of what she called "feeling colors." These colors may not be the ones that are typically attributed to an emotion, such as red for anger or blue for sadness. Rather, they are highly subjective and personally meaningful and even regulating, to the extent that children and adolescents may choose to wrap themselves in a large swath of silk in their chosen shade, or in the colors of the rainbow. Such a large bodily gesture helps in sensing, as well as seeing and communicating, emotion.

She described how in her drawing, "yellow is happiness," while movement into yellow orange in the same drawing showed a sensation and emotion that "began to be upset." As the color shifted to red she said it looked "frustrated and angry" (Richardson, 2009, p. 115). The containment offered within the boundaries of her artwork offered a calm space for reflection and alleviating distress. "You know," she said, "the colors . . . they are all different feelings." She began to sort through my box of rectangular beeswax crayons, which have saturated color and a wonderful scent from the beeswax. "Yellow is happiness" she said, "and the white one is happy . . . the gray one is somewhere in the middle. The light orange is a little upset, dark orange is mad, and the red one is frustrated and angry." The darkest green, she said, "is hardcore sad, when you're really upset with someone." The two blues, she noted, look like, "loneliness," and the darkest brown strikes her as "losing hope." The black, she said sighing, "is really, really disappointed." While she drew, she pressed hard on her paper with the large beeswax blocks, zigzagging with wide and intense strokes. She then wiggled a thick red pencil in through a rip in the paper and pulled, creating an even bigger rift. She began to layer the colors, and then to paste her deconstructed pages together, restoring her image and integrating the emotions within.

One of the strengths of art making in therapy is the "potential for positive, creative development at a time when destructive and damaging behaviors are at their height" (Liebmann, 2004, p. 73). Adolescents describe their "inspiration" to create a picture, a story, or a song, and sometimes remind adults that this inspiration does not come on demand. The processes of creativity, communication, and coping with challenges are closely intertwined for adolescents with autism. Creative exploration, the exploration of self, and the communication supported by the therapeutic relationship allow adolescents to explore and master challenges in their lives.

Process-oriented art making can be very freeing. When the resulting imagery evokes a peaceful and restful place, or positive affect, revisiting the painting or drawing is an important coping tool. The images that emerge can be taken home and used for reflection and as resources for calming. These images can help adolescents to identify the daily events, comforting rituals, and sensory preferences that help support a sense of calm and lessen distress, increasing positive affect and a sense of self-efficacy.

As adolescents explore the expressive qualities of materials for creating art, or for play, they begin to know new ways of seeing and communicating. Both art materials and sandtray images may be chosen to create a strong image of themselves. They can use these visual representations to more clearly see themselves in relation to others, and explore the movement taking place in their lives. "Potential and possibility," as Lyndsley Wilkerson (2008) has suggested, "are not fully formed things, but are part of an ongoing process." Wilkerson described her experience of learning art from an adolescent artist with autism, Justin Canha, and suggested how their shared process of art making revealed a great deal about each of them.

One adolescent girl painted herself and her friends as flowers in a garden. She talked about how she saw her friends as forming a comforting, enclosing garden, each one of them different, in the midst of which she could blossom and be herself. Another girl, with some urging from the therapist, chose a large stone to be her anxiety in the sand tray. She liked to use the sand tray, "to explore my creativity" (Richardson, 2009, p. 217) but one day when she was clearly struggling, I persuaded her to choose a concrete representation of her anxiety and to put that in the sand. We talked about how the creativity she felt was a strength was there to help her. She began to work with, and around, the heavy stone she had chosen. The natural materials she chose helped her to slow down and to work with difficult emotions. Through her play she realized "when I put in all those things I didn't like, then I knew what I wanted to see" (Richardson, 2009, p. 217). She was able to add figures to represent the things that make her feel comfortable. Working with many shells, stones, and images from and of nature seemed to amplify her positive feelings. As she balanced her anxiety, she revealed her strengths.

Sandtray image choices described as being "like me," or as representing the self, range from superheros or trains, to mermaids or butterflies, all capable of moving with a sense of direction and encouraging new ways of coping with challenges. One girl looked into the sand tray she had created and focused on the central figure. She told the story of her sandtray world from the point of view of a mermaid, and said, "She feels . . . kind of how I'm feeling . . . and the fish are curious, they want to be friends. She's in charge of the ocean over here" (Richardson, 2009, p. 118).

Exploring a frightening dream, another girl created a sand tray that was initially disturbing to her. She intently focused on finding positive figures to add, and gradually her fearful response to what she had created shifted. By finding reflective images to add to the sand tray, she saw the appearance and mood of the entire scene transformed. Picking up a sparkling geode she observed, "they are like people . . . we don't see what's inside." Such depictions of self are suggested through the choice of materials, the qualities embodied by the materials, and the energetic presence of what has been created, evoking a response in both the creator and the observer.

The figures for the sand tray may also be modified to more accurately express the story the adolescent wishes to tell. This can mirror the feelings of the adolescent themselves.

One boy created a "time machine," driven by "fear," that was a marvel of energy, showing just how it was both exciting and scary to move through time and toward change.

Play or art making are both very sensory. Sometimes adolescents are less focused on the creation of an image and more engaged in sensory exploration and observing the process of change. When one boy was feeling stressed and did not want to talk, he decided that it would be okay to play. He declared, "I'm not going to put how I am feeling bad in the sand." Instead, he found a way of playing that was dynamic and sensory; touching, moving, and even blowing the sand into shapes. He created the process of "continental drift" in the sand, slowly and rhythmically allowing what he had initially created to change. He cleared away space to portray blue water, and then covered it up again, much like the flow of the tide. Sand rained down over trees, and rocks rolled away and returned. He was soothed by this activity, calmed rather than excited, and able to stay with the process without any self-consciousness. The scene, he decided, was taking place at the end of the day, and he said, "think of all the things winding down and going to sleep." He decided that the sand can always change and return again. These simple processes of moving and shifting the sand and altering the landscape of the sand tray can help adolescents to feel more comfortable coping with both strong feelings and engaging with serious ideas. "Using our imagination," as one girl suggested, can help a great deal in seeing, and then experiencing, thoughts and experiences in a different way.

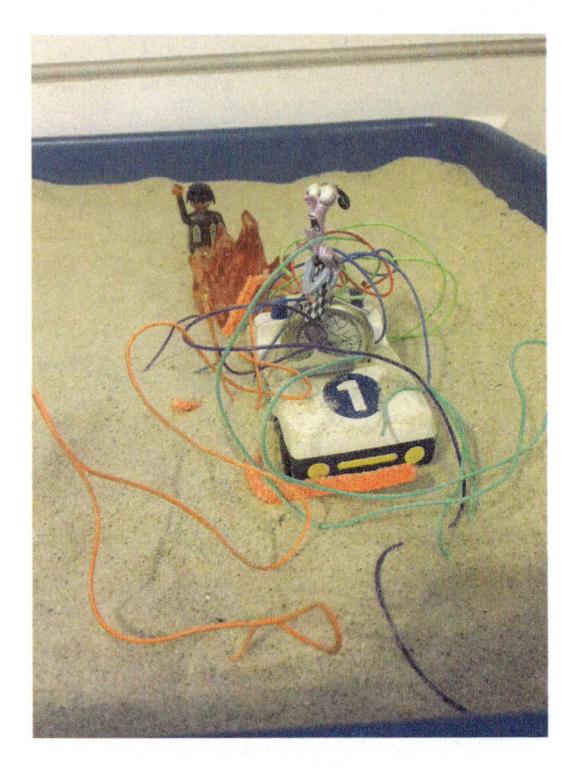

Figure 12.5 The time machine escaping a fire.

Sometimes this work begins spontaneously. At other times adolescents, particularly adolescents with a high degree of drawing ability or strong feelings of perfectionism, need considerable persuasion to work more freely, or even to draw at all. One boy loved drawing so much that he regularly carried drawing materials with him. But drawing was not always his choice in the context of therapy. We needed to find a form for his drawing that would allow the process to work for him. He settled on using very small paper, so that many images could be created and then turned into a small book. As he flipped through his series of images—things that he enjoyed, things that were funny, and things that were comforting—our conversation turned to the things he was thinking about that were more existential in nature. After creating comfort through drawing, he was able to raise big questions unrelated to his images, but made possible through their comforting presence. We discussed ways of coping with fears and how our thoughts could make us feel afraid. He suggested, "thinking about something else . . . that you like," might help him to feel better. He began to see how he could use drawing to help focus his own thought process to help him feel less anxious. Once such expressive and comforting processes are established, the range of challenges that adolescents can face in therapy becomes broader. While the feelings that arise while drawing are sometimes, as one girl described, "scary and sad," as Henley (2018) has suggested, "creative outcomes recognize the tenuous existential state of being their creator," (p. 81) and bring a sense of greater understanding and perspective.

Art making and play help adolescents to understand and master fears. Sometimes we see these outcomes through art. Moon (B. Moon, 2008) has discussed the important existential function of creating and reflecting on art in art, noting the power of art to hold deep and strong feeling. In the process of creating art work, or sandtray worlds, fearful ideation may emerge. Then adolescents are able to work on the relationship between thinking and feeling, exploring not only the fears themselves, but how actively doing something to address the fears, or to distract from fixating on fears, might help. Adolescents can take comfort from anxiety in creating balanced and structured patterns in their art, or in the sand tray, possibly in a configuration similar to a mandala. They often articulate how this process feels calming. One boy who struggled with depression and nightmares decided to work with a dream image that felt more positive, noting that the experience of creating this was like "infinite space," and comforting rather than frightening.

Once they have experienced an expressive and dynamic way of processing thoughts and feelings, adolescents are more open to exploring their lives and the world. Creating art or building a sand tray can bring a new perspective on thoughts and feelings, even feelings that seem overwhelming. One boy suggested that a black hole is scary precisely because it is all-consuming. Thinking about black holes made him think about human life and about our place within the universe. Playing helped him to depict his fascination and his understanding, and also to explore what is both alluring and scary about the vastness of space. He had not wanted to do this through making art, but eagerly gathered materials to fill the room with "the atmosphere, the planets, and the sun." Colored scarves, spheres of different colored minerals, rocks, and wooden balls formed the atmosphere, the galaxy, and the planets. Seeing, touching, and choosing from the natural materials in the space was an important part of this process. Choosing natural objects also helps to ground an "emotional connection to nature" (Kopytin & Rugh, 2017). For this boy, the choice of natural objects to portray a natural phenomenon allowed him to tell a story. A yellow physio ball surrounded by "gasses" made of silk scarves served as the sun. He filled the entire room with this installation. Then he chose a large sphere ball, which can open and close and swallow things up, to create a black hole. He animated the entire construction with great energy. At the end of this very active session, he looked over the universe he had created. He was able to see, and then to think about, how far away black holes actually are. He had taken his fear and enacted it, controlling the energy of the black hole. He realized, "I guess I don't have to worry about that so much."

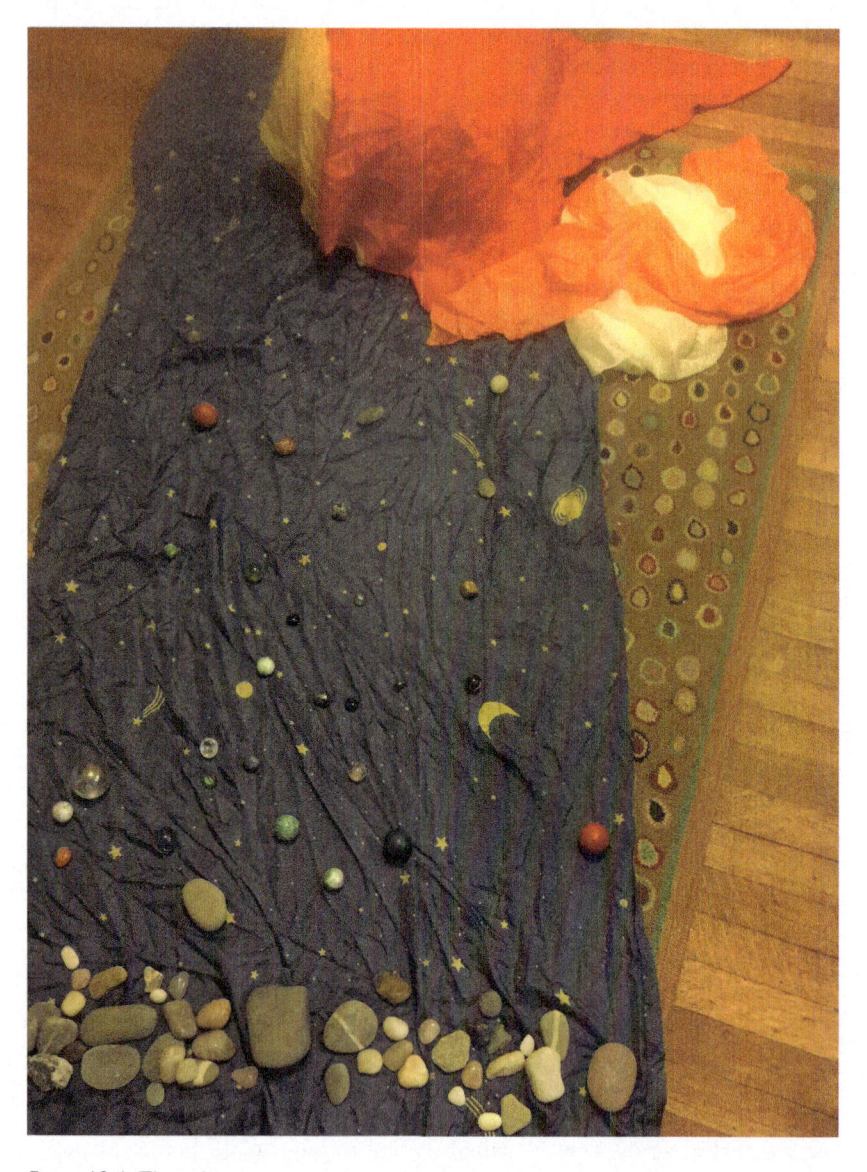

Figure 12.6 The galaxy.

For some children and adolescents, art making feels more familiar and comfortable than open-ended play. But playing can help even older adolescents to relax and explore different solutions to a problem. Sometimes playing with no agenda is challenging. Adolescents may feel stuck or uncertain of what to do, being drawn to play materials, but feeling uncomfortable in using them. One adolescent worked on ways to cope with worries and anxiety. We had some concrete goals and ideas that he had helped to generate, including identifying when he begins to feel uncomfortable, and using strategies that help with coping. He did a good job of identifying strategies that would help him, such as writing down worries, keeping track of what he has to do, and talking with adults as well as taking time to relax. He was so diligent about doing these things that he wondered if it was okay for him to be playful. As children move into early adolescence, play can be a welcome respite from increasing expectations and workloads at school. And yet, older children and adolescents may struggle with whether "it's okay to play," or whether the more mature thing to do would be "to talk about things."

I have seen an adolescent girl enthusiastically choose puppets, and then stop and look distraught, with one puppet on each hand. We established that this felt similar to when she becomes stressed at school and "doesn't know what to do." I asked if she wanted me to join in. I took two puppets and practiced getting one puppet to observe the other and respond to what they saw. I then explained "I didn't know what the second puppet was going to do! That's why I made him watch the other puppet first." These were my dragon puppets, a large one who breathes fire, and the small one who can't yet do this, "but would like to." I made the small dragon stick out his forked tongue but still not be able to do the same things as the big one. The little dragon got very frustrated initially, but my observer remained interested. We talked about what I had just done in my turn with the puppets. I suggested this playing was like "improvisation," where you watch—or in this case, where the puppets watch—what another person (or puppet) is doing to get some ideas for how to move or how to play next. Improvising, I explained, is a real skill, one that adults practice when, for example, they are playing music or dancing together. This "improvisational potential" (Brown, 2010, p. 19) of play helps the player to be more open to new ideas or new ways of doing things. Not only is it "okay to play," as one adolescent explained with relief, but contextualizing play in this way is important for those older children who might feel that play is "for little kids," however much they may be drawn to do it. We each took a puppet and practiced responding to one another, gesturing, waving, and tail wagging. Playing and improvising, she agreed, can be a good thing to do "when my brain gets stuck."

Play can be very focused with adolescents. They are able to use the process to explore transitions, decisions, and the emotions and relationships that impact these changes. One high school aged boy used the sand tray to explore his feelings about the transition to a new school, and how he hoped to learn

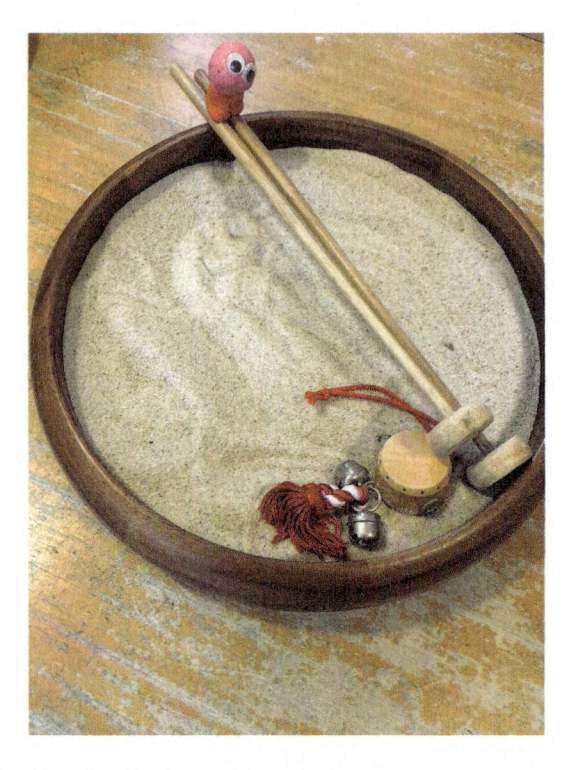

138 Potential and Possibility for Adolescents

Figure 12.7 Looking ahead in the sand.

more music, and to connect with others through music. Another used the sand tray to explore decision making about which activities to participate in, carefully adding to the sand every possible enjoyable activity to counterbalance the things that were sometimes both required and less enjoyable.

And a young woman used the sand tray to explore her transition after graduation from high school and her goals for the future, visually and viscerally presenting the forward movement in her life and her hopes for the future.

While adolescents with autism are working to understand the perspective of adults and peers, they also need to have their perspective understood by others. By adolescence, young people with autism often have developed greater observational skills, skills that can help them in perspective taking and in setting boundaries with others. One boy used actual fences to delineate comfortable boundaries with a peer. His friend was not good at respecting the boundaries of others. I was struck with his understanding of what the other boy needed. He talked about his relationship with his friend, who could be

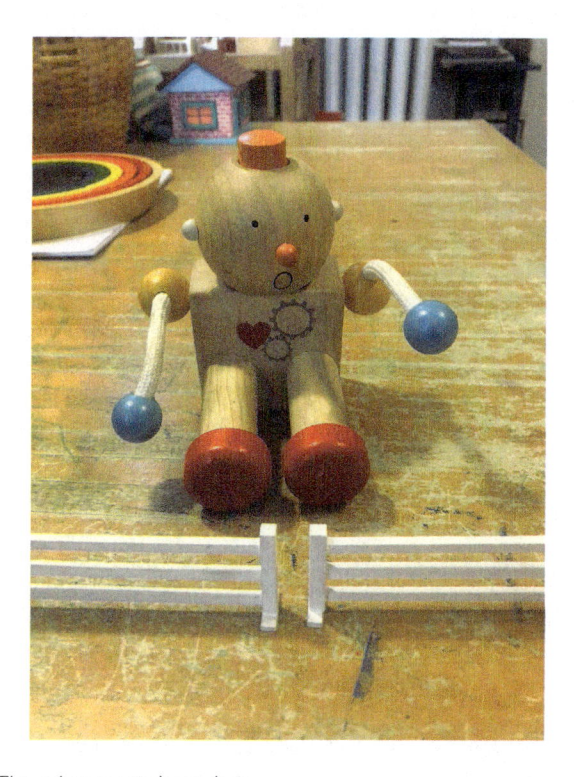

Figure 12.8 The robot meets boundaries.

demanding, even though, he said, "he understands me," and they share many experiences. He chose a robot figure to be the friend, who encroached on the personal space of others, taking whatever he wanted, from snacks to exclusive attention. Then he found a way to create a physical boundary, building a fence with a gate around the robot.

Adolescents need to understand that this creative and playful process is also productive.

Sensory materials sometimes help adolescents engage with making art, playing, or talking. A girl sitting on my soft blue sofa held a velvet pillow full of beads that she moved and stroked with her hands as she talked about her feelings of anger, sadness, and disappointment. We were not making much headway in our conversation, even though it was her idea to "sit and talk" at the start of the session, after choosing the pillow for comfort. I suggested that we try making some art. I suggested that we could work on connecting with who she is inside and what ideas she might have that could help her now.

For adolescents, the therapy space and materials for art making and play can "be apprehended instantly as belonging to another realm of experience" (Fox, 1998, p. 77) that allows for self-exploration. Adolescents experience this possibility in an increasingly mature fashion. Access to a creative space can help them experiment in gaining both freedom and control. But they need to be ready to enter into this space and engage with the process. One autistic adolescent girl described her communication through art as "thinking of and paying attention" (Richardson, 2012, p. 110) to the image she is creating. She then explained how this attention leads to greater self-understanding. Active work with materials and focusing images takes the immediate focus and pressure off of the individual. Therapeutic engagement on kinaesthetic, sensory, and imaginal levels creates space to explore feelings and thoughts.

The young woman with the pillow agreed to move from the sofa to the art table placed between two long windows, lit by the late afternoon sun. Once settled there, she said she needed a snack to give her energy before beginning to work. We took out some apples to share, and she noticed that "inside the apple, there is a star." She decided to try printing with the apple. I hoped that that simple image might be fun to make, creating movement in the feeling of "stuckness" she described. I realized that the print would create a mandala-like star pattern; she had been drawn to these images before, creating them in drawings and in the sand tray. She chose to print with yellow tempera paint, "like the sun." She became calmer as she laid out a sheet of paper, saying, "I feel good" as she smoothed it with her hands, and then became animated as she created prints for both of us. Revealing "what is inside" takes on a new dimension for adolescents. As they engage with the potential of their materials, and with the depth of their images, ideas and feelings are articulated more fully for others to see, and revealed more clearly to the adolescent themselves. Recognizing that their own imagination and sense of creativity can be a source of understanding and insight leads to a more positive sense of self, and supports adolescents to explore relationships with others.

One boy reflected through his art and in his storytelling how friends can help one another to find their strengths. He created two friends, one very tall, and one very small.

Together they discovered the things they both liked. He told their story this way. "They both like pancakes . . . they met at a pancake place. And they both ordered twenty pancakes. And then they found out that they both live in the woods." Together they opened a pancake restaurant, and found a way to deal with someone "who was not nice," building a house where "they could walk around in their yard and in the forest. The mean guy didn't have a key to the house. Only their family and friends had keys." Once they joined forces to win over the "mean guy," who was jealous of their success, he apologized for being mean. The story, he explained, "shows you can be friends with people no matter how different they are from you."

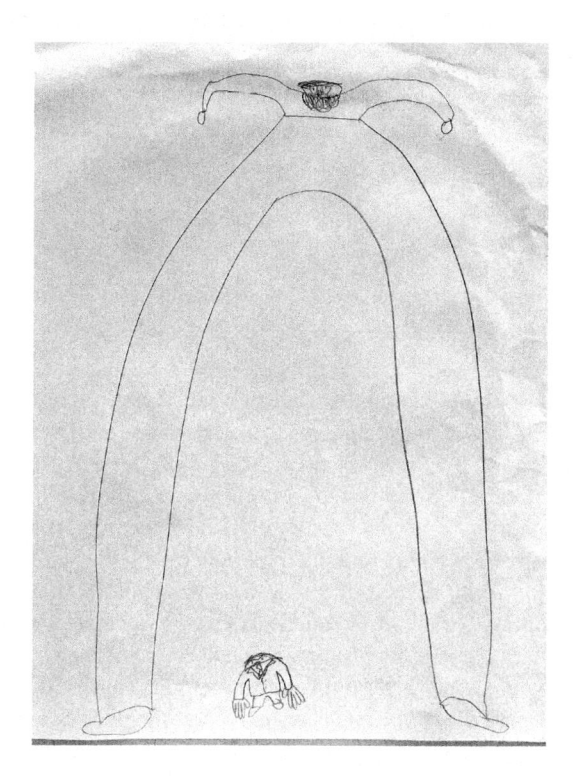

Figure 12.9 Very different friends.

Chapter 13

The Spectrum and the Continuum

The expressive therapies continuum (Lusebrink, 1990, 2016) is a developmental model of how emotional, sensory, and movement-based interactions with art materials and art making processes support expression, integration, and deeper understanding and insight. Lusebrink conceives of how the continuum moves from a foundational sensory and kinaesthetic preverbal level to an integrative creative level. Art making experiences, even at the simplest level of the continuum, such as painting with fingers or rolling clay, can take on meaningful richness for the artist, and thus provide a creative experience. At early developmental levels, as Proulx (2002) describes, "the process becomes the symbol" (p. 164), moving from engagement with materials and processes to meaningful expression. The experience of creating gives rise to an affective state of receptivity and calm.

As they create art, children are exposed to pleasing or integrative sensory activities, gently increasing the range of what is pleasurable to them in a natural way. In her work with very young children, Proulx (2002) has discussed the way in which she advises parents to follow "the developmental abilities of the child" (p. 17) as a guide to an unfolding creative process of playful, sensory-based shared art making. Evans and Dubowski (2001) describe "a freer and more relaxed relationship with the art making process during art therapy" (p. 10) for children with autism. This is in marked contrast to what they may experience in an art class, where there is pressure to produce a finished product. Relaxation of the pressure to produce results allows the kinaesthetic experience of art making, and the sensory qualities of materials, to be explored in a nonthreatening way. While creating art, children may experience new and integrative sensory experiences as well as developing their personal style of visual expression. While a child is working, the therapist attunes to the child and takes into account the child's rhythm of working, level of comfort, and style of communication, both verbal and nonverbal.

Current perspectives on autism recognize the biologically based connections between the brain and the behaviors seen in autism. Herbert (2012) notes that autism "involves the whole body," (p. 7) the mind, and the brain. Miller et al. (2015) have discussed how "process-based," relational multisensory interventions help children to form connections and become more regulated (p. 153). Grandin (Grandin & Scariano, 2005) explains how "my tactile senses were overly sensitive . . . but my kinaesthetic senses were wide open for learning" (p. 151). When individual sensory preferences are understood, working with responsive and flexible materials and processes encourage flexibility in the child, and exploration of new materials can lead to increased expression. One child began covering a previously popped sheet of bubble wrap with lots of intense and splotchy red paint, excitedly saying, "It looks like blood!" As he continued painting, his strokes of paint slowed down, and he began to add other colors, all the while breathing more calmly and focusing on the image as well as the action of painting. The gesture and the color transformed this simple printing plate, which then revealed "a rainbow" as the color transformed and he appeared more relaxed.

While art therapy builds on the visual strengths that may be present in autism, therapists also need to be sensitive to these sensory aspects of creating art, which are not primarily visual. As he observed children responding to art, Burri (in Vecchi & Giudici, 2004) noted how, "We experience our reality through our entire body just as much through the pores of our skin as through the retinas of our eyes" (p. 33). The experience he describes, that of taking in the visual world through the medium of the body and the senses, is also present in therapy as we create and share art.

Through the process of art making, children may be exposed to pleasing and integrative sensory activities, increasing the range of what is pleasurable, and even regulating for them. Hinz (2009) suggests that experiencing the shift to this calm inner state is in and of itself a creative act, since a child can "bring forth something new (a relaxed state) as a result of the sensual use of materials, such as flowing color on a brush" (p. 7). Schweizer et al. (2014) explored the importance of "offering varied materials and opportunities for expression to enable various kinaesthetic, creative, as well as sensory means to communicate" (p. 14) for children with autism. Prizant (2015) recounts how for those with autism, there can be "joy derived from the combination of the feeling of the material" (p. 36) and an understanding of and communication about the material.

Kranowitz (2006, 2018) discussing the needs of "sensory children" with processing differences, emphasizes that these children need to FEEL materials, with all their inherent properties of flow or resistance. Children with heightened sensory needs, explains Kranowitz, when they are oversensitive to touch, "will avoid touching and being touched and will shy away from messy play . . . on the other hand, if they are under-responsive to touch sensations, they'll crave touching and being touched. These children will be fingerpainting their arms!" (2018). The materials a child or adolescent with autism will respond to most fully are mediated by sensory sensitivities. For example, as Bogdashina notes, when a child is seeking sensory input, "they often yearn to interact with a variety of tactile stimulating objects"

(Darewych, 2018, p. 318). Other children, who may be avoiding more sensory stimulation, may prefer to work in silence, or reject materials that are textured or scented. As Bogdashina (2016) has observed, the sensory and perceptual worlds of autism are unique. Although, she suggests, "autistic people live in the same physical world and deal with the same 'raw material' as neurotypical people, their perceptual world turns out to be strikingly different from that of non-autistic people" (p. 55). Sensory preferences and sensitivities, as Grandin has described them, are "at the core of autistic experience" (Silberman, 2015, p. 425). Thus the sensory and perceptual nature of both art materials, and of art making processes, are important considerations in therapy at all developmental levels.

Challenges in regulating emotions may color autistic children's responses to experiences, to art materials, or to the other people who present or participate in these activities. Children who become overstimulated by the effort required to focus attention on what they are doing and remain responsive to others may feel confused and fearful, becoming visibly anxious or withdrawing into behavior they find soothing. Children may also experience extreme sensitivity to environmental stimuli, whether sounds, smells, or textures, or the presence of other people or particular objects. Their sensory responses may be so acute and uncomfortable as to be completely disorienting. In this situation, there may be difficulty in sharing space, activities, or even, as Henley (1992) observes of working in the studio with autistic children, sharing "the same field of vision" (p. 70).

For children whose strengths may be more visual than verbal, the social pragmatics of communication may prove mystifying, leading to difficulty establishing mutually satisfying relationships. Art making provides an opportunity for children to communicate through making and sharing art, as well as, or instead of, talking about what they have made. This communication process engages the child in a reciprocal, relational process that Prizant (2006) calls social communication. Social communication includes the ability to participate through, and communicate about, mutually satisfying shared activities. Among the skills required for social communication are joint attention abilities and symbolic behavior. These are skills that are strengthened through art making, where children are able both to attend to activities and materials and to communicate symbolically. Wetherby and Prizant (2000) describe how social communication supports children's growing abilities in a variety of ways, noting that children are more fully able to share both their intentions and their emotions when they engage more comfortably with others. Their ideas, intentions, and emotions can then be communicated through art and through play. The individualized SCERTS model for supporting autistic individuals focuses attention on the interrelationship of social communication with emotional regulation, facilitating these therapeutic goals with "transactional support" (Wetherby & Prizant, 2000) that is physical and sensory as well as emotional and communicative. When using art, play, or other expressive approaches with autistic children and adolescents, transactional support from the therapist may include modification of the environment or materials in addition to supports for stress, anxiety, and coping that allow for exploration, expression, and communication.

Art making can then build on the strengths seen in autism, when therapists "partner to develop symbols and better communicate ideas" through "shared creative experience" as Goucher (2012, p. 296) describes. And as Rubin (2005) explains, this communication is a developmental process, unfolding as art making is explored in a relational context. Gray (2002) has described autistic children as moving more fully into "the complex dance of reciprocal social communication" (p. 4) through shared, meaningful activity. When we make art, we also enter into a relationship with our materials. Moon (B. Moon, 2008) has described how this relationship is equally essential to the art therapy process, and explains that, "multiple experiences, such as tactile, visual, and procedural ones, simultaneously occur in art therapy. The intersections of relationships and experiences are where the curative aspects of art therapy are enacted" (p. 117).

Materials, as McNiff (1995) suggests, are evocative. This is true whether they evoke a sensory response, an emotional response, or the creation of an image. Dolphin (2014) has discussed how the inherent *potential* of materials is fundamentally important in offering a multitude of possibilities for communication, creation, and relationship. Open-ended and natural materials alike offer great freedom for transformation and improvisation. Art making is a tactile as well as a visual experience. Tactile and spatial challenges may come into play when children explore, or are reluctant to explore, the art making process. Vecchi (2010) has described how a child new to painting has first to, "deal with being confronted with a large, white sheet of paper, making the first brushstroke . . . entering a relationship with this empty, unknown space" (p. 110). Art making becomes a particularly interesting "crossroads" for children with autism, as Martin (2009) describes, "because it is an activity in which strengths (visual learners, sensory interests) and deficits (imagination, need for sensory control) merge" (p. 28). For example, a child exploring paint may become excited or they may become frightened. Vecchi (2010), while not describing a child with autism, has captured this balance between engagement with, and fear of materials. She describes how "the material/color that with 3 year olds often gets transferred from paper onto hands can be a disturbing and unwanted presence for some children, and they need to be certain it can be washed away and that their hands go back to their original state" (p. 110). When they begin to make art, children may need reassurance. They want to know that the color they have chosen is expressive and beautiful, and not only "messy." It is a revelation to understand that paint will move, and mix, and change, but that it will also define their space and their image. Children need to feel that the experience of painting, despite not being entirely under their control, can be enjoyable.

When art materials are used in therapy, they must be considered within the context of the therapeutic relationship. Children learn to trust the process of working with materials through the support of this relationship. Within a relationship, they also learn to communicate about both the process and what they have created. Using materials to enable communicative language requires what Wadeson (1987) calls an aesthetic choice, a personal choice that considers the needs of the individual and the unique significance of their images.

The Nature of Materials

Art therapists sometimes define materials and media by their influence on the art making process (Lusebrink, 1990). Media are identified as fluid and likely to evoke emotion, or solid and likely to evoke internal structure during the creative act. Kagin and Lusebrink (1978) have categorized materials from fluid to resistive and discussed how the medium influences both the image and affect. Generally speaking, "fluid media are likely to elicit emotional responses and resistive media are likely to evoke cognitive responses" (p. 32). Martin (2009) discusses these properties of materials in relation to the sensory profile of children on the autism spectrum, noting that materials need to be chosen or presented in ways that are inviting and not overwhelming. Children and adolescents may find their own way to work with materials, and their own relationship with them. Therapists, as Orbach (2020) cautions, need to allow themselves, "to observe, to wonder, and not to control" (p. 14) the child's unfolding relationship with materials. The environment for art making needs to feel safe, and, as Bogdashina (2016) describes, others must try "to move in the same sensory world" (p. 235) as the child, enabling them to make choices and feel a sense of connection.

For people with autism, sensory responses to materials are connected to individual ways of processing and perceiving. Grandin (2016) has discussed various ways of responding to the world that also correspond to an individual's response to materials. The categories of processing she discusses are: visual processing, auditory processing, touch and tactile sensitivity, and olfactory sensitivity, all of which might be related to how an individual experiences particular materials as pleasurable or not (loc. 1238). Bogdashina (2016) suggests that adults need to know "how children experience the world through each of the sensory channels, and how they interpret what they see, hear, and feel" (p. 116).

Children have strong materials preferences. One little girl, who loved to create solid, three-dimensional work, searched through the baskets in my art closet and exclaimed, "How did you know I loved cardboard?" Of course, she also enjoyed the process of cutting or tearing the cardboard, the texture of the board, and even the sound of ripping. She was not put off by the faint smell

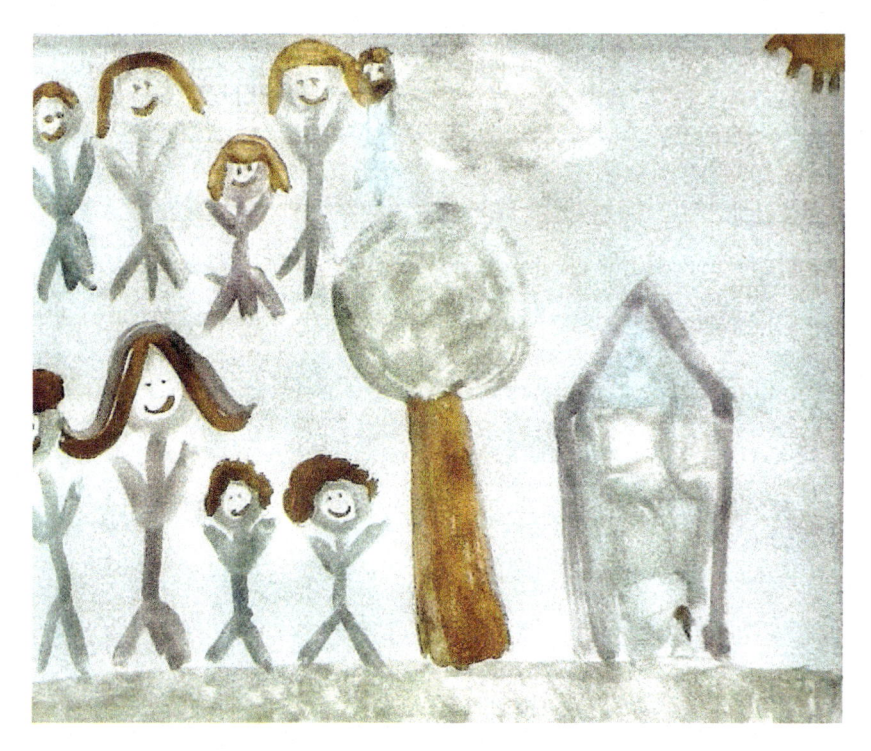

Figure 13.1 The glowing family.

of the layers as she ripped across them. Other children like only smoothly moving crayons, made with beeswax or soy wax, and still others like only fine point markers. They use these carefully chosen materials to realize their vision of what they want to create. Treffert (2013) notes that in making art with people on the autism spectrum, therapists often find, "skills consistent with unusual sensitivity to various sensory stimuli, superior visual memory . . . and innate access to what has been called a 'picture lexicon'" (Treffert, 2013). One young girl used this sensitivity in choosing which paints to use for a portrait of her family. While her style was very simple, her choice of luminous paint colors gave the entire family a glow that could be felt by the therapist as well as the child. She was able to portray both her family members and also the way in which they were important to her. The creation of this image led to a discussion of the people in her family, and how they are all different, and special to her.

Traditional art materials such as paint require both sensory engagement and physical gestures to create imagery. Digital media provide an alternative means of accessing and creating personally meaningful visual images, and they can be very appealing to people with autism. Many children I have worked with enjoy creating and sharing animation and videos around their interests and original stories, even when they also might enjoy using the traditional two- and three-dimensional materials available in my art room. Using digital processes can engage individuals with high sensory sensitivity when materials requiring more sensory engagement are not comfortable. Virtual tele-play or art therapy with autistic children or adolescents makes a necessity of exploring digital processes and children's interest in digital media in a responsive fashion. During the COVID-19 pandemic, the children and I experimented both with hands on play and drawing that we shared digitally, creating digital images, and a blend of the two. In a mix of hands on art making and digital communication, we created portraits of one another by tracing over the image of the other on our screens, and embellishing these drawings as the subject or the artist requested. Children became minions, space explorers, or major league ball players, and they portrayed their therapist as part of their digital, as well as their social world.

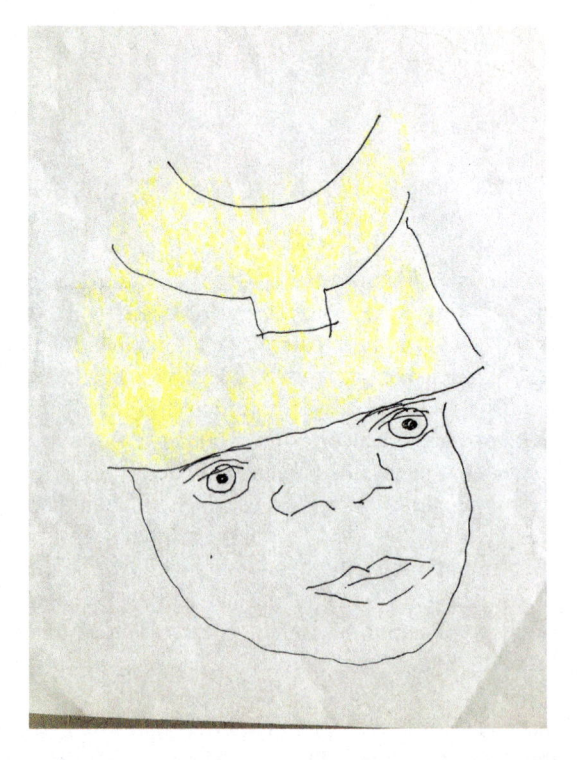

Figure 13.2 Portrait of a child made by tracing the face on the screen: "turn me into a minion."

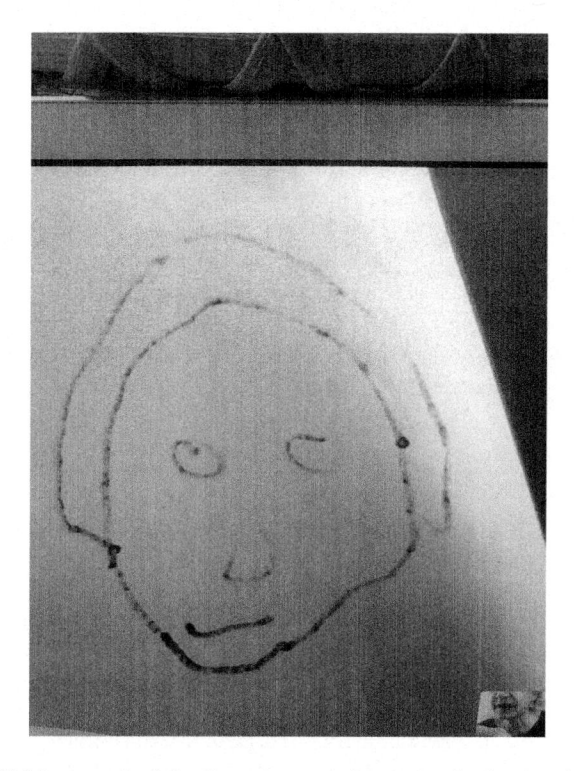

Figure 13.3 Child's portrait of the therapist, made by tracing the face on the screen.

In face-to-face therapy, Darewych (2018) found the use of painting apps to be one nonthreatening way of creating work that still connects with significant experiences and relationships, and enables communication within the therapy session. While working with responsive and flexible materials can encourage flexibility and exploration, the primary goal of working with any material is to support increased expression and communication. Maintaining the balance between engagement with materials and comfort with expression is essential to creating art in therapy, whatever the nature of the materials that are used.

Different materials bring out different feelings and different possibilities. While the calming or energizing effects of drawing, painting, or shaping clay can be alternatively soothing or enlivening, this is not always the case for children or adolescents with autism. Therapists must always be respectful of children's individual rhythms and interests, and they must be flexible and responsive in ways that may not have occurred to them until meeting a particular child. For many children and adolescents, the process of creating art fulfills a sensory need, but it may also present sensory challenges. Therapists need to know both the child or adolescent and the materials, and they must choose the materials they present carefully. The presence of the therapist supports the exploration of materials. Through the shared use of these materials, images become an expression of interests, ideas, and feelings. Most importantly, this presence supports the therapeutic relationship, enabling growth and change, and attuning to individual preferences and rhythms. Hosseini (2012), in surveying the work of artists with autism has observed how "due to an intense desire to cut, to tear, to blend colors, to put sticks and other materials into their works, individuals on the autism spectrum are naturally drawn to their unique, preferred art form" (p. 10). Working with materials to discover their inherent expressive qualities, and developing personal themes through art are therapeutic processes that help children to communicate, self-regulate, and grow in self-awareness. Creating and sharing images helps, as Mullin (2015) suggests, both to engage with the world and to "filter" the world (p. 16) both through individual perceptions and the sensory and physical process of art making.

The Developmental Process and the Expressive Therapies Continuum

Each level of the expressive therapies continuum is seen to have a distinct function, and the movement through these levels supports both greater expression and an unfolding sense of self. Art therapists, as Moon (C. Moon, 2010) notes, "explore how different materials specifically help expression at different levels" (p. 40) of development. And Robbins and Sibley (1976) suggest that there exists a "psychology of materials," whereby "each material has a capacity to activate a unique response in the user" (p. 136). Through observing children carefully, it is possible to see what Vecchi (2010) has described as, "child and material in dialogue together" (p. 33). Therapists are able to support this essential dialogue for children and adolescents with autism through varying materials and processes to widen the experience of art making in a playful and pleasurable way.

Lusebrink (2016) discusses the continuum's various levels as engaging both hemispheres of the brain in integrative and developmentally based ways. People making art, whether children or adults, move toward a more "integrated functioning" (p. 61) both through the use of materials and the creation of images. Creative experiences, she notes, are possible at any level of the continuum.

At the foundational kinaesthetic/sensory level of the continuum, children need to experience themselves in space and in motion before they are ready to create marks or images. Developmentally, this is the preverbal level where experience is rhythmical, tactile, and sensory. Young children need lots of practice in handling materials. Their mark making may not initially be intentional; rather, they may bang on a piece of paper, or run with a marker touching a roll of paper, and then discover to their delight that they have made a mark.

There is a sense of satisfaction in learning, as Miller (1989) has observed of autistic children, "to translate body actions intentionally into marks on the paper" (p. 302). Materials must be responsive enough for children to see the evidence of their movements in the marks they create. A large expanse of paper on the wall, as used in the Miller method for autism, can help a child to see marks that appear as the result of walking or running with a drawing instrument. Subtle differences in materials are important here. A therapist working with Miller's approach noted how, "I used markers that were very responsive to pressure so that even the slightest pressure left a big mark on the paper" (p. 309).

Kinaesthetic experiences, such as pounding clay or tearing paper, can be energizing. They can also be soothingly repetitive, as with quietly spreading paint, or repeating a shape through drawing or printing in a rhythmical fashion. The rhythms produced can also create entrainment (Kossak, 2015; Hinz, 2009), a synchrony of rhythm that is calming and particularly valuable in autism, as this internal sense of rhythm is relaxing and comforting.

For children with extreme sensory challenges (Gabriels, 2003), regulation through the senses may be a focus of therapy. The sensory qualities of materials, especially very responsive materials such as clay or paint, may be calming and focusing. Autistic children can experience manageable and pleasurable levels of sensory experience through art making. Evans and Dubowski (2001) discuss using this satisfying element of the art making process as a foundational base for the therapeutic relationship in art therapy. The sensory/kinaesthetic level of the continuum continues to be particularly significant for those with autism. What Bogdashina (2016) describes as, "the qualitative nature of sensory experiences" (p. 58) are always individual, and they remain present, and important, at all developmental stages.

Exploring materials on the sensory level can develop into the creation of images. Lusebrink (2016) suggests that simple motor-based expressions with materials can manifest shifts in energy as well as indicate the beginning of imagery. And, as Hinz (2009) discusses, the "emergent function" occurring from sensory stimulation results in an increased awareness of the affect that is generated while creating. For example, as Lusebrink (2016) has suggested, slowing down movement may increase the ability to focus on sensations, and to communicate about them. One young adolescent loved creating creatures that could move. He experimented with clay, finding a way to intricately hinge together, and thus articulate, the various body parts of his beasts and birds. While these creatures were astonishing in their detail, and beautiful to behold, they did not completely satisfy his sense of movement. He was able to slow himself down, and accept all of his creations in the process of exploring their movement. Then, incredibly quickly, he colored paper to fashion into a flying bird that, while it had less detail than his carefully rendered clay creatures, moved swiftly and gracefully, fulfilling his need for movement as well as his vision.

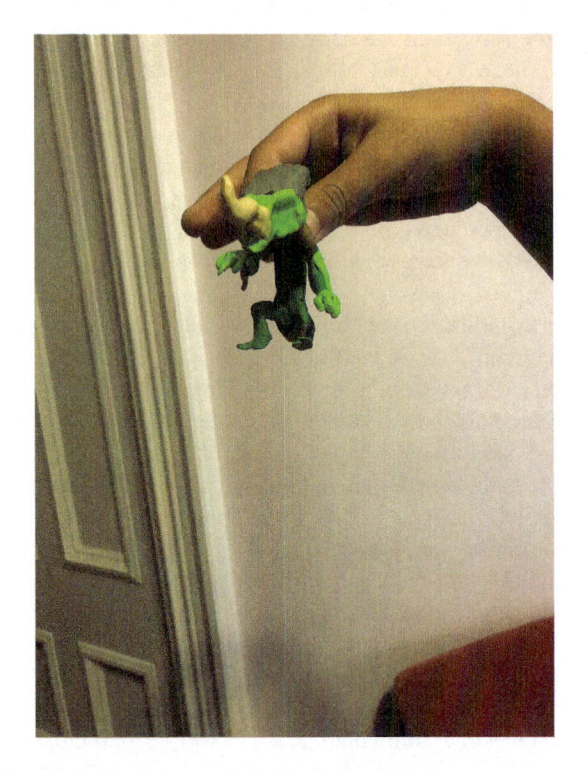

Figure 13.4 Articulated creature made from air dry clay.

Sometimes, however, children will be drawn to materials that Martin (2009) describes as (p. 71) "matching," rather than soothing, their sensory state, and too much of this can be dysregulating. Van Lith et al. (2017) discuss how it may sometimes be appropriate to work "top-down" (p. 82) through the expressive therapies continuum for children with autism. Beginning with the child's highest level of ability both acknowledges and supports the integration of new skills. This approach may also address gaps in development by beginning with materials and sensory experiences that allow the child to feel a greater sense of familiarity and mastery. Many children I have worked with prefer initially to use black crayons or fine point markers, which offer them a sense of control both over the flow of the material, and the clarity of the final image. This autism-specific way of working remains sensitive to the importance of materials and art making in building the therapeutic relationship, and, as Van Lith et al. (2017) note,

> Despite the often bottom up implementation of the ETC, the continuum model provides flexibility for working top-down, bottom-up, and within

fluid approaches. Working in a top-down fashion through the ETC addresses . . . gaps occurring in the development of individuals with ASDs.

(p. 82)

To this end they suggest using structured materials such as markers initially, before moving to more fluid or messy materials, which children with autism may initially refuse, or even feel overwhelmed by. Some children who feel more comfortable beginning with marker or pencil may wish to exclude color from their drawings entirely. When they have successfully established that they are able to draw, and portray a preferred image or theme in a way that pleases them, then they are more willing to experiment with new materials, processes, and playful approaches.

One adolescent girl who had a great deal of mastery of drawing materials preferred to use familiar materials that she could control. She created striking self-portraits with pencil, successfully sharing the qualities she chose to highlight, and allowing her to reflect on these aspects of herself. Painting in watercolor on wet paper was initially scary to her, but ultimately rewarding. She felt the satisfaction of feeling and watching the flowing paint, but also that of having created an image of a landscape. Her painting both conveyed the feeling of a place she enjoyed, and gave her a sense of calm as she reflected on her work. Her experience is an example of moving through the different levels of the continuum with a fluid, integrative approach. While she had moved well beyond the sensory kinaesthetic level of development, she still was able to benefit greatly from the experience of using more flowing, less controllable materials; and she was able to appreciate the very different imagery that this made possible.

Another potentially frustrating, as well as rewarding, material is clay. Clay requires movement to create form. Clay requires physical energy, and sometimes tools, to work. The effort required can feel just right, helping the child to connect to the process of creating or to the therapist, who can work with clay alongside the child, or create a figure to interact with the one created by the child. Henley (2018) describes how "staying hands on" (p. 22) helps children who are either distracted or extremely active to focus enough to communicate with the therapist, or with others in a group. The continual movement and incremental change inherent in working with clay may connect with a sense of playfulness for some children, even as it engages their attention and allows for sustained focus.

Clay may feel too difficult or overwhelming for a given child on a given day. On my art table there are two small wooden containers, one filled with kinetic sand, and one with "floof," which is like very soft and fluffy white snow. Children sometimes choose to run their hands through one of these materials, watching them shift or rain back down into the container. Or they may try to impose more of a form on them, making a "sandcastle" or a "snowball," or even more complex forms such as a small house, even though this is not their intended use. To create a shape from these materials takes minimal hand strength, focus, and time. Sometimes children want to play with what they have created, and sometimes they want to linger in sensory investigation that they find calming and satisfying. When they feel comfortable, there is an opportunity to move toward using more permanent materials, such as clay, to create an image that is more lasting. If children can make this transition, their effort is rewarded with a more permanent figure, one that they can paint and keep, and alter to look more like their vision of what they wanted to create.

While the kinaesthetic process is engaging and compelling, as Martin (2009) has observed, children, or even adolescents, with autism may also get "stuck" in repetitively exploring or using materials. It is then difficult to move on to representational work, or sometimes to any work that they wish to communicate about. This is why, at the appropriate point, scribbling, like investigating sensory materials, sometimes needs to be guided and supported as part of a developmental process. The "scribble chase" (Hinz, 2009; Malchiodi, 2003; Malchiodi & Crenshaw, 2014) is a scribble-based interactive process that is initiated by the therapist. With children this becomes a game, where the therapist, or the parent in a joint session, begins drawing a line that is "chased" by the child. While simple, a great deal is taking place relationally during the scribbling. As Malchiodi (2011) explains, the awareness of the other's movements, marks, and presence during the scribble chase supports attunement with the other, and also flexibility in the child. Hesitant children can become engaged in this shared drawing as it is very clear what they need to do: follow the therapist's line. All they need to do is choose a color. The adult and child mirror one another's movements, and fall into a shared rhythm, within which they can feel felt, as well as seen, by one another. Osborne (2017) describes such interactive processes as a "window of rhythm" (p. 17) within which we can connect to one another without words.

Many children enjoy being the leader, with the therapist following, or with a parent or sibling when the scribble chase is introduced in a family session. Following first, and learning from the therapist what to do, enables children to then take the lead. While this is a kinaesthetic activity, the expectations are also structured and clear, and children rarely decline to participate.

The next step of the drawing process is to find images in the scribble, and to make a picture out of them. While finding and elaborating on the images, the child and the adult are creating meaning and a story together. Drawing together rhythmically is an example of what Athanasiou and Kharkou (2017) describe as nonverbal "proximal communication" (p. 274) that supports relationship.

Such a shared art making process helps children move sequentially through the levels of the Expressive Therapies Continuum, as Hinz (2009) has suggested. Working on the foundational kinaesthetic/sensory level (including, sometimes, smelling the markers or other materials), with its strong sense of movement, progresses to the perceptual/affective level when images are identified and elaborated upon. Some children are able to create a story about their pictures, and others are not. Storytelling would move this activity to the cognitive/symbolic level, a shift that children do not always make. Hinz (2009) notes the importance of supporting shifts between levels in creating greater flexibility. Sometimes I have found that the "story" of the images created is played out nonverbally in the sand, or with toys or images on the art table, rather than through talking about art work.

Other forms of kinaesthetic art making that engage the body on a large scale, such as body tracing, may seem intrusive to autistic children, as it might breach their boundaries (Martin, 2009), whether of sensory comfort, or the interpersonal boundaries needed to maintain personal space. When children can comfortably create this larger scale of work, there is often a relational story to be told. Drawing on a large surface creates images that sometimes mirror back feeling in a way that is easier to "read."

One approach to large-scale mark making is the "interactive window" devised by Miller (1989). This window provides a large vertical plexiglass drawing surface which stands between the child and the adult. The parent or the therapist draws together with the child, as they watch and respond to one another's movements. When the child is engaged with what they are seeing in the "moving picture" the adult creates, the child becomes both "interested in producing that pattern," and also more interested in the person who is making the drawing with her (p. 313). Miller has noted how such shared drawing experiences support the growth of relationships. He also observed how children grow in awareness of their parent when they draw together, and describes how, "it makes the mother a moving picture . . . it has made her watch her mother . . . her whole awareness of her mother is different . . . and she looks at her much more" (pp. 312–313).

The second developmental level of the continuum is the perceptual/affective level. Expression at this stage may or may not be accompanied by words. Images may be emotionally charged, and express an emotion, or alternatively they may show attention to formal elements of art, however simply these may appear. This is the stage where children begin to express their understanding of the world through drawing. Their drawings are individual, expressive, and emotionally rich. Portraying and sharing perceptual experiences are one way of beginning to understand the perspective of others as well. During the developmental stage correlated with this level, children are using forms to portray their felt experience of the world as they observe it. For children with autism, who may be absorbed by drawing, and have a facility with this visual language, drawing becomes an important form of communication. Work done on the perceptual/affective level may not always need words to communicate meaning. Children express their understanding of the world through their drawings, as Lowenfeld (1975) observed. For autistic children, as Martin (2009) explains, shared art making, and observing the art of another, is "akin to hearing their point of view" (p. 71).

Drawing with a child also develops the use of the art therapist's third hand in relation to the child's way of drawing. The therapist may alternatively be scaffolding the child's willingness and ability to draw, or to use a new material. Or, the therapist may be learning the distinctive approach of a child, like the autistic eight-year-old who advised me, "one thing you could do, is go slow around the edges," his description of a sensitive way of drawing slowly enough to feel the shape of the object being drawn.

For another child with a clear and inflexible sense of the "rules" for our sports-inspired play, I had the constant challenge of his intolerance of any "mistakes" I made, usually in the form of a breach of the rules of the game. One of our tasks was to find a way to play together, and to understand one another's perceptions of and perspective about what was taking place in this play. Given that my knowledge of rules and statistics in baseball, basketball, and wrestling was far less encyclopedic than his, I would make mistaken "judgment calls" during our play that could be distressing for him. I suggested that we create some trading cards together, an activity he enjoyed. He often grabbed the *Inside Out* figures to play with, introducing them into his sports- themed play in the sand tray. "Anger" was always out of control, whether it was his turn to run bases, shoot baskets, or wrestle. While he created very detailed images of basketball players on his cards, I decided to use the *Inside Out* figures to make some cards from a series I titled, "Feelings and Wrestling." When we looked at one another's drawing, he decided that I had made a "new series" of cards, never seen before, and certainly not available in stores.

We observed how "Fear" could withdraw from the match, where "Anger" might be carried away and be as ineffectual as he was strong. Our shared art making carried our shared play forward, to a place that was less repetitive and more interactive. He began to see my perspective, as someone who didn't know as much as he did and was trying to learn new things. We traded cards, since he was eager to take my images home. Shortly thereafter, he brought me one of his own much-loved wrestling figures as a gift for my sandtray collection.

Hinz (2009) has observed that, "work with the Perceptual dimension can help clients begin to perceive themselves and their world differently," noting that "what can be perceived in an image can perhaps be more easily managed in real life" (p. 89). This child's ability to share, to manage frustration, and to moderate anger all grew through the use of this play and these images. Perceptual experience of the world is different for people with autism, as is their sensory experience. Bogdashina (2016) describes how while "autistic people live in the same physical world and deal with the same 'raw material,' their perceptual world turns out to be strikingly different from that of non-autistic people" (p. 53). Sometimes, to help children feel more open to experience, we need to work with their preferred interests and images in a new and more reciprocal way.

The Spectrum and the Continuum 157

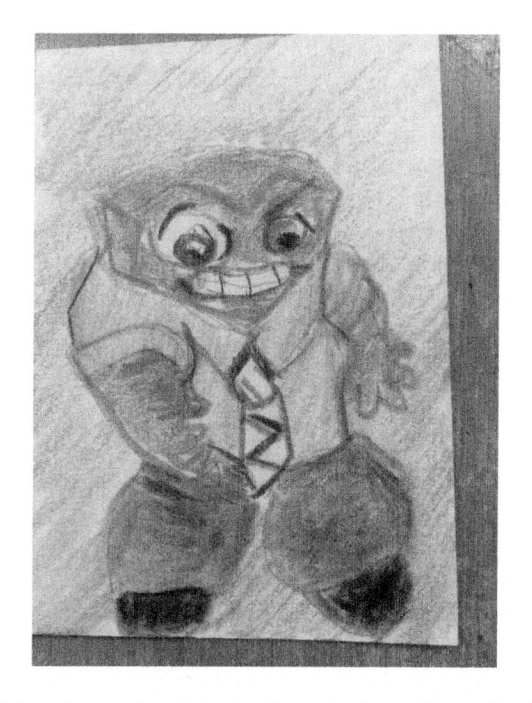

Figure 13.5 Artist trading card made by the therapist: "wrestling and feelings."

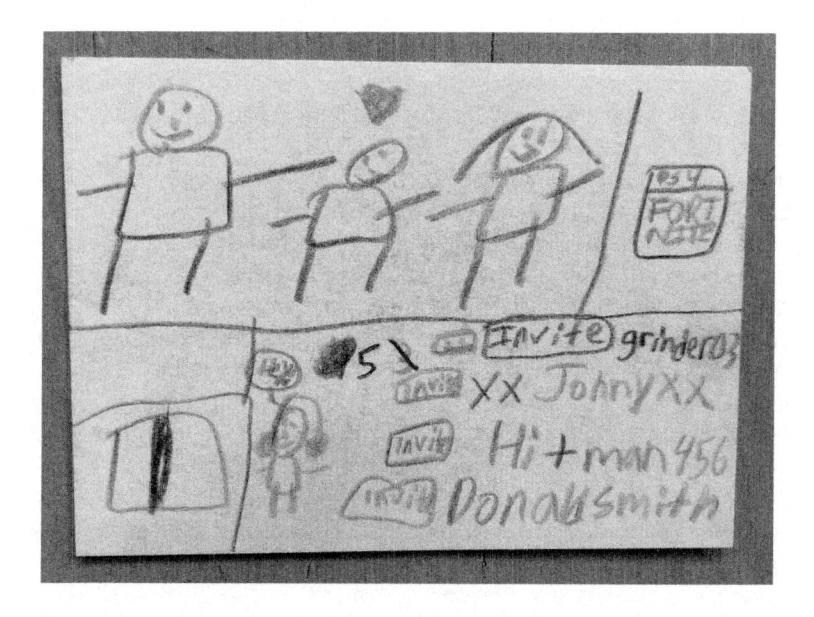

Figure 13.6 Trading card of wrestlers made by a child.

Children can be helped to look at the world of others, and at their place in this shared world in a clearer way through making art. One child who had persistent problems attending in his classroom, in part because he felt so uncomfortable at his place at the table, was able, at the therapist's suggestion, to draw a picture of everyone's physical place in his class. He depicted himself looking distressed and crowded by a child with whom he had trouble getting along. When this drawing was shared with his teachers, with his permission, the teachers immediately perceived how stressful this place was for him—something they had not yet observed—and a change was made. He was able to feel more relaxed, attentive, and positive during the school day as shifting his physical position in the room was accompanied by a shift in his experience of the room as a social environment.

As at the kinaesthetic/sensory level, children can seem to be "stuck" at the perceptual/affective level, copying or creating images repetitively. The challenge in working with autistic children is to consciously work with these preferred images in such a way that we encourage communication and flexibility. The images and the stories that may accompany them thus become more dynamic, because they help the child to share their experience, and to then move forward in communicating their experience. One child combined drawing and sandtray play in a story about a train. The theme of the story was taken from a much-loved movie, but the faces were created by the child to affix to my wooden trains. He depicted an engine being withdrawn and parked inside a tunnel, and not wanting to come out. After taking a break, and when he felt comfortable, the engine changed his mind about wanting to be with others. This story was similar to the child's own hesitation about participating in events with peers. The faces he created were very expressive. Looking at and playing with these images made it possible to touch on the affect generated through this play. Drawing and playing helped the child to think of ways he himself could feel more comfortable, and more ready to join in activities he was curious about.

Kramer (1979) warned that therapists should not move children away from their familiar, comforting images too quickly. This is certainly true of children with autism. Sometimes conventional, or even stereotypical images represent a needed defense against internal chaos or confusion. Children's preferred images can be used to build communication, and as Grandin (2015) says, gently widen restricted interests. Hinz (2009) describes how art therapy uses "a visual language as a parallel process to their verbal communications, to differentiate and depict their internal experiences, thoughts, and emotions" (p. 98). Creating and reflecting on art work can literally help children to see more clearly, with greater awareness of emotions and experiences.

The third level of the continuum, the cognitive/symbolic level, corresponds to the ability to think more abstractly, and to understand experiences outside of personal experience as meaningful. At this level, there is more planning of the art making process, and more intentionality behind the work. Children, and particularly adolescents, are increasingly able to conceptualize their experiences visually at this stage. One adolescent portrayed her friends as a garden of flowers, nodding and moving and receptive to her. Looking at and creating this sort of expressive work can be affirming and enlightening. At this stage, art making is a way of consciously addressing a challenge or a confusing situation. Therapists help to support this process by suggesting ways to elaborate on and develop art work over time, such as making a series of drawings or a book. Once a challenge is contained visually, it can be addressed, and changes over time can be observed together.

At the far end of the continuum—the creative level—elements from all the previous levels become integrated. Sensory engagement with materials, the perception of forms and their significance as they emerge, and planning for intentional creation all have an important role at this level. Art work takes on deeper meaning as a personal expression or symbol. Creative experiences, believes Lusebrink (2016), have the potential to integrate both hemispheres of the brain, and they can also take place at any level of the continuum. One example she gives is particularly meaningful for autism. She discusses how "a sense of calm can be created without the formation of an external image: the media experience itself can induce serenity" (p. 30), even with a simple material. Through engaging with materials, an art object can be created that engages both the mind and the body. This balance of mind, body, and senses is present in non-Western views of the creative process, which can help in understanding the role of creativity at all levels of development.

The Creative Level and the Flow of Creativity

The idea that art making and the rhythmical flow of energy are intertwined is essential in the philosophy of Chinese art, and in the work of non-Western arts therapists (Richardson et al., 2012). The fundamental principle of Chinese painting, as I learned when I first visited Beijing for the Creative Arts Therapy Conference in 2011, is the visual expression of the movement of life and energy of the spirit (Van Briessen, 1998). From the Chinese perspective, working with energy in therapy means engaging with art but also with the whole person: the mind, the body, and the senses. McNiff (2011) has discussed how "creative expression is given the freedom to move according to the immediate and infinitely variable conditions of a person's life," and Ross (2011) suggests that making art both engages the emotions and restores the flow of creativity.

Werner (2012) explains how creative engagement is possible on many levels of experience. His developmental stages, as in the Expressive Therapies Continuum, begin with the fundamental importance of the senses and of movement. Werner describes the sensorimotor-affective level as a level of experiencing where young children do not clearly differentiate themselves from the outside world, feeling a unity between the self and what is perceived. At this level, children are aware of things being separate from themselves, but are more selectively attentive to the things they feel connected with. But even when children and adults reach the level of abstract thought, he believes, the richness of earlier levels of perception can still be available to them, together with the ability to integrate these levels in a creative way.

Werner called this ability to access earlier, more sensory-based levels microgenetic mobility. He was interested in how children move through the different levels of development (in Crain, 2005) and also how mature development, and more fully developed expression, is enriched by the sensory, kinaesthetic, and perceptual experiences that first arise at earlier developmental stages. This ability to move through different developmental levels is a process that integrates both primitive and more complex forms of thought. Such movement through different developmental levels is a process of integrating the sensory and the kinaesthetic with more complex forms of thought. The perceptually based, movement filled, sensory experiences typical of earlier levels of thinking and perceiving serve, at higher levels, to connect the senses, the emotions, and cognition in a creative synthesis. According to Werner, this mobility and richness is most fully accessible to artists. My Indian colleague, Shaloo Sharma, describes how she has seen this sort of movement and sensory awareness throughout the working process of autistic artist Anshuman Kar, noting how, "he just loves the touch of colour on paper" while creating his strong imagery. She explains that, "he is absolutely relaxed while painting and I can see that his hands are flowing, and his strokes relaxed" (Sharma, 2020).

Children, as do artists, explore materials, connecting their imagery with what is seen, felt, and ultimately, shared. They respond through sensory, kinaesthetic, and perceptual exploration of the world, finding ways to represent their understanding of, and their feelings about their personal worlds. This is why Picasso (Ashton, 1988) famously said that it is so important, and so difficult, to draw like a child.

Some autistic people with savant skills are able to readily access earlier levels of memory and experience, and to use this access across levels of development in their creative work while moving freely across levels. Bogdashina (2016) discusses memory in artists with autism, and how "privileged access to their memory allows them to produce outstanding results in art" (p. 135). The work and working process of autistic artist Michael Tolleson Robles offers a striking example of how the creative interplay of movement and memory becomes integrated, and then manifests through his painting. At age 61, he describes himself as "a true autistic." He is a self-taught, savant artist with a flourishing international career. He has had the experience of "plotting," as he describes it, his "own way within the art community—a journey from my soul and my creative abilities" (personal communication, January 16, 2019).

Before he began to paint, Tolleson Robles found "I did not find my light in myself." Rather, he explains, he found "154 ways to camouflage myself," in an effort to fit in. Art became a way for him to explore situations and emotions, and also a way to "open dialogue" with others, in such a way that he now feels "the art socializes for me" (personal communication, January 16, 2019).

"Where the art comes from?" He explained, "I have no idea." For years now, he has been able to "funnel into art . . . who I am, what I represent, a persona." He then added "art that speaks has emotion." He shared his view of how a painting can contain and "reflect all of us," including "despair, disappointment, strength," through an image that becomes both a "container for creation" and an emotionally charged image. "The dialogue of a painting," he said, "is my voice" (personal communication, January 16, 2019).

He explains that when he began painting, he had an idea of what it was like to be an artist, and he knew how to immerse himself in painting. He explains how "when I paint, everything shuts down, and I only know the canvas and the paint." And yet he found what was most essential was that "I went back to my roots. I went back to my child. I try not to lose the child." Because he was so completely engaged in his work, he was able to create "the wild and crazy piece, true to the child within ourselves." He reminded me that when working with children, adults must "always see through the child's eyes" to support emerging strengths and communication (personal communication, January 16, 2019).

Tolleson Robles is very clear about the continuing significance of process in his work. While he often works in a series, he explains that his subject, for example a boat, "is a subject, not the process." In one of his boat paintings, he may be more focused on the "quality of the water" and the resonance of the work as a whole, always asking "Where's the spark. Where's the spontaneity?" (personal communication, January 16, 2019).

Autistic artists have ways of thinking, of perceiving, and of using sensory information that makes their work especially strong and vivid. Tolleson Robles explains how "I see color within color within color." He described an experience in middle school, while working with pastels and being told by his teacher, "there's no purple in the shadows." This was a direct contradiction to his perceptual experience. "At that time, at that age, I SAW that," he explained. Now, as an artist, he continues to connect to such acute perceptions, freely working with his direct experience of color to "do what feels right. A blue shadow feels cool and right." He reflected on his personal palette and how paintings "convey feelings and emotions" through color as well as through the image. And still, he observes, "I had it all along." He had that heightened awareness of color and the ability to bring this perceptual immediacy to his work. For an artist with autism, there is no other way. As Tolleson Robles explained "we can't create filters that don't exist" (personal communication, January 16, 2019).

The relationship of art and autism, as Tolleson Robles describes it, is integral and fundamental. He describes how his process of painting "happens within the autism," and he feels that "I have to get away from it before I see it." When I asked him his thoughts about Werner's concept of microgenetic mobility, his answer suggested that this process was at work in his perceptions, and his art. The painting, he explained, "presents itself to me." His perceptual cues to create the image, are not yet "conceptualized . . . I don't know what it will look like. I'm a vessel, and the autism paints" (personal communication, January 16, 2019).

Chapter 14

Experience Becomes a Doorway: A Parent's Story

Based on Interviews With Jennifer Damian

The arts provide a place where the imaginative and social worlds converge. Experiences in the arts support expression and the growth of self-awareness; they can also form a base for shared experience and deepening relationships. Art images represent, as musician and mother Jennifer Damian describes, "the truth of your experience" (personal communication, April 19, 2012). For Jennifer's son Kai, who was diagnosed with autism at the age of one year, visual art, music, and dance have all been an integral part of his life, providing languages for expression, communication, and growth. As Greenspan (1996) has suggested, "The child can develop a rich inner life only if she has experiences from which she can derive and refine inner images" (p. 84). These inner images, represented through the arts, can reveal the self to others, perhaps especially so when people create together.

Therapists who use the arts in therapy have much to learn from other contexts in which the arts are practiced and shared, including the families of artists. As a middle school student, my own son wrote an essay for admission to an intensive arts program, which he titled, "Home Is Where the Art Is." He talked about growing up not only with an awareness of art history far beyond what he had learned in school, but with the creation of visual art present as an active part of his environment and of his own development. In a family, as in an arts community, the arts can provide a "natural support," as described by Leonora Gregory Collura (2012a) for a child with autism. For a classically trained musician like Jennifer, the arts can "set the mind into motion" and provide focus, while also "opening doors in your mind to the bigger picture around you" (Collura, 2012a).

As the mother of a child diagnosed with autism, Jennifer wondered how her lives as an artist and as a mother would be intertwined, and if she would ever be able to share her music with her son. She remembered the heartbreak of the singer Beverly Sills, when she learned her own deaf child would never hear her music. Jennifer wondered if Kai would ever be able to watch her perform, and be able to hear her music. She had no way of knowing whether Kai would ever, as he has today, "experience what I experience" through music. From her years of teaching Jennifer had extensive experience with students with special

DOI: 10.4324/9781315173306-14

needs, and her training as a musician helped her to "see creative possibilities around situations" (Collura, 2012b). Jennifer was also aware that while the arts allow for expanding creativity and curiosity, and an increased opportunity to perceive the world in fresh ways, they simultaneously provide structure that can be regulating for children. This broad understanding of the role of the arts in learning helped her to find ways of sharing the arts with Kai. She hoped to be "as open as I am in music" (in Collura, 2012b) as she supported her son. She saw possibilities for integrating arts experience with structured therapy goals, when parents, therapists, or teachers see and take advantage of creative opportunities and approaches informed by the arts.

Jennifer wanted to share her own experience with Kai, and felt lucky that as he grew, "he saw enough like I did" (J. Damian, personal communication, April 19, 2012) to engage with dance, visual art, and eventually, with music. Kai saw his mother engaged with music, and saw her communicate with others through her art. For Jennifer, the base of understanding through the arts provides a structure for a parent, teacher, or therapist to offer communicative, expressive, and integrative opportunities to children.

Jennifer had the experience to understand Kai's sensory profile, which included unusual sensitivity to sound, so much so that even the sound of the ocean would be distressing to him. Some genres of music were completely overwhelming to him. And yet, as Kai grew up, as Leonora Gregory Collura (2012a) observed to his mother, "everything you've experienced in your life, you've opened up for your son." As a baby, Jennifer found a pattern of rhythms to use with Kai that he found soothing, first sharing this as a touch-based rhythm on his back. As he got older, Kai was able to mimic his mother and to play the rhythm she was playing on a drum. These shared rhythms built relationship and attunement with one another.

Immersion in a creative process has been a natural way of learning for Kai. His mother's understanding that the arts "open doors in your mind to the bigger picture around you" (J. Damian, personal communication, April 19, 2012), has helped to shape this picture for him. She explained how the goal focus of a practicing artist, coupled with the necessity to "take direction from an outside source—the arts," (personal communication, April 19, 2012) can help children to assimilate both a structure and new skills. At the same time, they are encouraged to be flexible, expressive, and responsive.

While his mother was introducing him to music and the arts, Kai was receiving intensive sensory-based therapies with music in the background to help acclimate him to the sound. Greenspan (2012) has explained that it is the "daily work of gifted parents that makes gains possible." Building an individualized program to address the neurological, communication, and sensory challenges of autism was a daunting task. Jennifer recalls how, "each specialist had their own theory of how he would or would not develop" (Collura, 2012c). Kai began speech therapy at sixteen months. He also worked with physical therapists and occupational therapists to address sensory integration challenges. His mother's guiding principle in building his program was to "look at Kai's personality" (J. Damian, personal communication, April 19, 2012) as well as his needs, and to build a therapeutic environment that was holistic and nurturing. A cornerstone of this therapy was Greenspan's DIR Floortime (Greenspan & Wieder, 2009), which builds attunement and communication between caregiver and child. Without Floortime in particular, his mother felt that Kai would be a different child, not reaching the potential he has attained today. The language Greenspan uses to describe the process he innovated is very resonant with Jennifer's integrative and arts-based approach. Greenspan (2012) has spoken of how therapy goals include helping a child "become more creative and more expansive." The Floortime (Greenspan & Wieder, 2009) approach to working with children and parents is built upon careful observation of a child, "tuning in to her interests, emotions, and goals" (p. 93). Engaging a child in two-way communication involves incorporating a child's interests or activities into the communication process. Greenspan offers this example: "if a child is dancing around the room, a caregiver can offer a hand and see if she'll take hold of it, and the two can dance—now it's a two-way dance" (p. 84). Through the relational, interactive process of Floortime, Jennifer saw Kai became more regulated, calmer, and more connected: more "expansive" in many dimensions, to use Greenspan's description of the process. His progress also allowed for the introduction of new experiences; since, as his mother reminded me, best practices of autism support and therapies do not leave a great deal of time for other activities.

Having begun with Floortime, his mother introduced what she described as "modified, naturalistic, ABA" (J. Damian, personal communication, April 19, 2012) therapy, which offered more choices to Kai than a stricter Applied Behavior Analysis protocol. Always, she was aware of neuroplasticity, and the developmental window for helping Kai build greater flexibility, communication, and integration. Working to extend these possibilities for him, Jennifer said, "with this knowledge, I became very intense about what was out there" (in Collura, 2012c), providing intensive therapies and also biomedical interventions to address physiological challenges such as allergies and gastrointestinal symptoms. With intensive therapy, Kai's sound sensitivity dropped, but he still avoided his mother's music. Porges (2011) has identified a group of children with autism who are acutely sensitive acoustically, and Kai appears to have been one of these children. The discomfort from such heightened sensitivity, Porges has noted, may be perceived by children as threatening, and even as detrimental to engaging socially. Wisely, his mother did not push Kai into music, but offered other experiences in the arts. All of the arts, in Jennifer's view, have the potential to help children replace core challenges with new skills. She realized that music too had the potential to make him "very happy" when and if he was ready.

Kai began a ballet class for children with special needs at the age of five. He also took part in Joanne Lara's dynamic Autism Movement Therapy, a neurologically based and highly interactive creative movement approach. I met Kai and his mother while doing my own training in this integrative approach. During classes and trainings, students, whether they are children or professionals, all became immersed in the process together, learning through repetition, attention, modeling, and eventually sharing. As Joanne Lara describes the guiding principle of her work, "AMT is an empowering sensory integration strategy that connects both the left and right hemispheres of the brain" (personal communication, March 3, 2012). The careful progression of Autism Movement Therapy, feels Jennifer, has "made his brain a little more open" (J. Damian, personal communication, April 19, 2012). I observed Kai being first a partner and then a leader of other children in his movement class.

AMT is actually designed to redirect processing, building on children's potential through the repetition of sequenced movement patterns, and integration of the different senses. Children see the movement patterns, hear the music, and use their bodies to respond. Joanne Lara explains, "everything you have to say comes through the body . . . the body is able to speak when the mouth cannot" (personal communication, March 3, 2012). When they are ready, and their kinaesthetic and emotional awareness of one another enables them to do so, the group of children shifts to constructing stories or poems to be depicted later through movement. This multisensory and integrative approach, Lara explains, "helps individuals with autism in processing, storing and retrieving information in a more efficient and effective manner" (personal communication, March 3, 2012) that is then available to them to access more freely in everyday communication.

After watching this process unfold for her son, Jennifer has come to feel strongly that, "without dance, you would have a very different child" (personal communication, March 9, 2012). Movement and ballet, Jennifer feels, are each structured to provide a "clear, organic structure for learning" (personal communication, April 19, 2012) that allows children to understand what they need to do: first feel the movement, and then to succeed in moving in a way that communicates and connects with others.

Kai has built friendships connected with each of his arts activities and settings, engaging with friends who have different levels of ability. In the Autism Movement Therapy group, I was able to observe the connection between the children, who seem to notice one another's nuances and preferences for movement, and when they are more experienced, to build on these in their own movements and sharing. Jennifer agreed, and explained how the children have come to know and accept one another's personalities, both paying close attention to one another and being calmed by one another. They support and encourage one another, "paying tribute" as Jennifer observes (personal communication, March 3, 2012) to one another's successful shared expression, and building on one another's energy. As the children come to understand the intention behind one another's movement, it is possible that, as McGarry and Russo (2011) suggest in their discussion of the role of mirror neurons in dance therapy, "one important route to emotion recognition involves a neural simulation of another person's emotional actions in order to infer the intentions behind those actions, and empathize with them" (p. 178). This process of "mirroring" is also considered "to enhance emotional understanding and empathy for others" (ibid). Mirroring can involve the imitation of movements or the communication of emotion through movement. For Kai and his friends, sharing movement, art, and stories has been a way to build stronger relationships and greater empathy.

Lara's Autism Movement Therapy works through combining patterning, visual movement planning, auditory processing, rhythm, and sequencing through "a 'whole brain' cognitive thinking approach, that can significantly improve behavioral, emotional, academic, social and speech and language skills" (Lara, 2016, p. 1). Creative and interactive approaches, as Greenspan (2012) felt, are "not so much work for the child but a challenging new experience that leads to mastery." New experiences can help wire the brain and provide opportunities for growth.

A sense of emotional security coupled with this sense of engagement and reciprocal communication is the "deepest foundation" (Greenspan, 1996, p. 41) for addressing the neurological challenges of autism. And Siegel (2012) feels that the emotionally resonant dimension of interpersonal communication is critical to our ability to experience close connection and emotional regulation. He suggests that, for children with autism, we need to create what he calls, "growth promoting interpersonal connections" (2012, p. 317). Both Greenspan and Siegel suggest avenues of connection to a child that are open ended, responsive, and playful. In Jennifer's words, this playful, arts-based connection to a child is "making the brain a little more open."

In facilitating this process, "words," suggests Siegel (2012) "are often quite limited in their ability to convey our internal states. Attunement to one another's nonverbal means of communicating emotion is a much more direct and satisfying way to join with others" (p. 181). This is particularly true for children with autism who are experiencing challenges in verbal communication. For these children, as Siegel (2012) suggests, we all "may benefit from keeping an open mind about creative strategies for helping introduce and maintain growth-promoting interpersonal connections" (p. 317). These strategies must originate in our response to the child, as Jennifer's experience with Kai and music illustrates.

Although he has perfect pitch, Kai avoided music until the last year. Jennifer describes how, "My son who said he hated music wanted to join a choir" (J. Damian, personal communication, April 19, 2012). After watching "The Choir" on television, Kai was riveted to every episode, and then told his mother that he really wanted to sing in a choir. Jennifer described how this inspiration and enthusiasm came about for Kai:

> There is a man named Gareth Malone—he is the conductor of BBC's "The Choir" and also a very strong music educator. He is young and he

has worked with the London Symphony and many other musical groups. He has that ability to turn around the learning to a positive stance in basically everyone he meets, but especially including children with disabilities. He is full of knowledge about how the arts become a platform and a doorway to learning in each child. He truly inspired Kai to want to sing in a children's choir, and feel safe doing so. I think that show made a huge impact on Kai's view of music, as it supported what I had been showing him on the sidelines for years. I believe that because it was from an outside source—one who believed the same sets of values about the arts and education as I did—Kai took that to heart.

(personal communication, April 19, 2012)

Fortuitously, there were auditions the next day for a children's choir, where the directors were looking for the children's awareness of pitch and rhythm, both strengths for Kai. He was chosen for the choir, and later given the chance to perform with them together with the LA Opera.

All the early musical experiences his mother gently introduced to him created a feeling of safety with music. This sense of safety is essential to allow strengths to flourish and become a base for learning, connection, and self-expression. Awareness of the need for safety is essential in our providing children with what Leonora Gregory Collura (2012c) has termed, "the right mix of support and development" for an individual child. Awareness of strengths can become a cornerstone of self-awareness.

Both Kai and his mother ride horses and have a shared love for animals. Kai has done therapeutic riding, and the family has had beloved dogs, who were an essential part of meeting early physical therapy and occupational therapy goals. His sensitivity toward and attunement with animals helped his therapists to attune with Kai, who was calmer walking with his dog. This dog had a personality that sensed when Kai was going to cry, or needed calming, and her inclusion in therapy created a calmer and more natural environment for therapy.

Kai also developed a growing interest in tactile activities and crafts. Kai is now passionate about drawing what is important to him. He gained an ability to "focus on very detailed scenarios visually," (Collura, 2012c) and his mother gave him the opportunity to take art classes, eventually joining in a summer camp for gifted children where his mother taught. As he became increasingly interested in visual art, Kai created many pastel drawings and clay sculptures of animals. As a younger child, who was "overjoyed to be around animals" (Collura, 2012c), Kai was introduced to clay as a preschooler, and happily fashioned creatures ranging from dinosaurs to dogs, working alongside his teacher who wanted to nurture his evident visual strengths. Immersion in this engaging material worked well for Kai. He created figures that reflected his feeling for animals. Kai learned from his teacher, who gave direction as well as offering flexibility; but he also learned from the material itself, working on his figures and finding, as his mother described, a way to "use his mind a bit more" (in Collura, 2012b) as the clay encouraged him to pull out images of his beloved animals. Leonora Gregory Collura, in her discussions with Jennifer, noted how Kai was able to communicate more fully through art. Each material he explored—drawing, painting, clay and pastels—seemed to engage him in a different way. His mother describes "wonderful autistic interpretations of how he saw the world" of animals (in Collura, 2012c).

His mother again observed his problem-solving process at work when Kai created a video game out of a box, designing everything from the game controls to a laptop computer, and creating them from cardboard. He became absorbed in the process and with his creation without any need to have prolonged play with the actual game itself. He was able to modify the potentially challenging situation of playing an electronic game into a creative, hands on response.

The opportunity to observe others creating work and to work alongside them has been inspiring for Kai as he matures. In the group setting of a collaborative "Art of Autism" exhibition, he saw older autistic artists "doing their own thing" (J. Damian, personal communication, April 10, 2012) in the art studio and was eager to draw alongside them. Within the studio environment, Kai encountered "a community of creative individuals who happen to have autism" (Collura, 2012b). This ability to "be in the art together" is akin to what Lara (personal communication, March 3, 2012) sees as the basis for all learning in the arts: the opportunity to be with and working alongside people who love their artistic practice. This is how children are supported by and learn from relationships as they learn from art.

Kai sensed the importance of creating images and objects to the older, more experienced visual artists. He was intrigued enough by their process to follow through on his own. His mother describes Kai's awareness that the older artists in the exhibition were "doing their own thing, but passionately" (J. Damian, personal communication, April 19, 2012), not talking a great deal, but rather teaching by example. As his mother described this learning process, the exposure to mature work awakened Kai's curiosity. "It was," she described, an "exploding" interest in making art, that appeared to have been "dormant within him, and suddenly a door opened and he was expressing" (in Collura, 2012c). For Kai, the arts have provided a place to access the community around him and build friendships. Art offered him a starting point for personal exploration and the opportunity to be immersed in art with others. As Kai watched autistic artist Joel Anderson at work in the studio, his mother suggested, "Why don't you paint with Joel?" (in Collura, 2012c). She noted his initial confusion about where to start, but Kai was able to pull out a sketchbook and begin drawing. His mother described him later "going into that flow" (in Collura, 2012c) in a way that felt natural to him, making a transition from watching others to creating himself in a calm and focused fashion. Jennifer suggested that a central question for parents, teachers, and therapists is to ask: "How can a child take in a new experience?" For her son, the response to this question reveals "awareness of who he is as a person, and who he is going to become" (personal communication, April 19, 2012).

Chapter 15
Conclusion

In therapy, very young children may choose to draw, paint, or play in the sand. They may speak a great deal, or very little. They may linger over sensory toys or materials, or dive into play and creation. Older children and adolescents also use the open-ended materials and processes of art and play to explore their understanding of themselves, though in a different way. Through the creative process of art and play they reveal their thoughts, their feelings, much of who they are, and who they are becoming. Art making may become a source of confidence, as they see themselves as able to create their own vision and share their own story. These experiences in therapy both reflect experiences in the world, and support broader, and more fulfilling, experiences and relationships with the others who are part of their world. As children gain flexibility and communication skills through therapy, their desire to connect with others, to play and share with them, can then be supported in the context of their community and their peers as well as within their families.

A preschooler settled Charlie Brown into the sand tray and declared, "I'm a good boy." While the figure in the sand was speaking these words, he was also reflecting his own positive new experiences. In the months since we first began to work and play together, his interaction among his peers had changed. After adapting to the routines and expectations of a new school, which provided a better fit for his needs, and as he became comfortable in his new environment, he was sought after by his peers for play. His increased communication made this adjustment easier for him, and feelings of connection were reflected in his play in therapy as well. He began to give attributes and feelings to the characters in his play, bringing friends together in the sand tray. "Hi Linus," he said, bringing a friend to be with Charlie Brown and interact with him. And he invited me to help explore friendship alongside him. "Make him talk!" he suggested, as the cast of characters for his play lined up along the edge of the table. I picked up a scared looking figure, and when I said, "I'm scared," making the little person shake a bit, he took this character from me and put him inside of the doll's house. "It's okay," he said, "I can be your friend." As children gain comfort and greater expressive abilities, they also experience

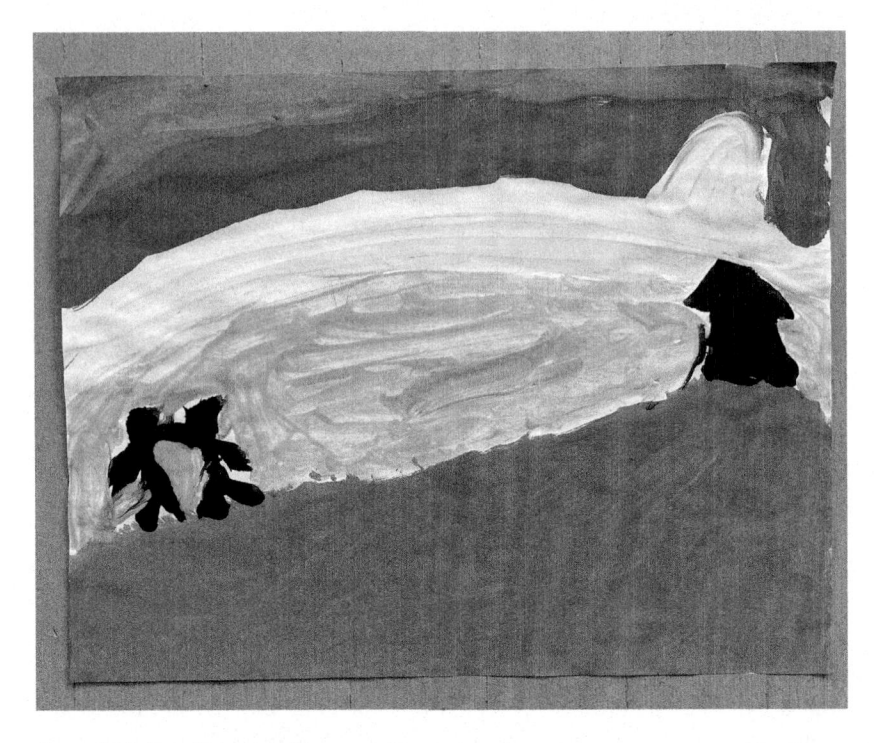

Figure 15.1 Two friends walking together.

themselves in a different way. They then bring what they have learned in therapy into their lives and relationships with others.

When therapists, parents, or teachers see change in children and adolescents, it is important to understand what has changed, and also to understand how it seems to have changed. The effects of playing, drawing, painting, or shaping clay can be self-regulating. Flexible materials for art and play encourage flexibility, even as they enable communication. Images can speak of both feelings and ideas. Playing and engaging with children and adolescents through their interests, and through their senses, supports their ability to tell their stories more fully through their art or through play. Noticing what has changed helps children or adolescents to appreciate how they have grown, regardless of how much they may verbalize either the process itself, or the changes that have taken place. Listening for the meaning of what we do not hear is as important as attending to words since meaning emerges from the process of play and the imagery of art. And yet spoken language may also blossom, as it did on the day when one young child introduced me to one of my puppets, beautifully practicing social communication and also offering me reassurance, saying, "Don't be scared . . . I'm a baby monkey! Hi Doctor Jane."

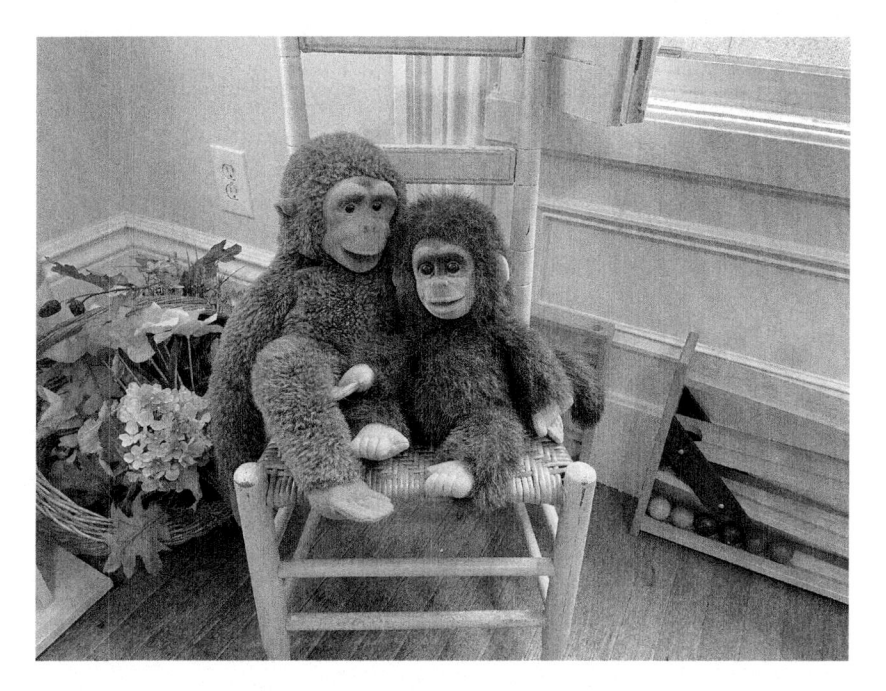

Figure 15.2 The monkey puppets meeting the therapist.

Across the world, in Delhi, a preschooler thoughtfully created an elaborate sand tray full of animals, deliberately choosing creatures that appealed to him and sending them into his world in the sand. Only at the very end of our time together did he choose, and add to this scene, two little boys, sitting together in comfortable chairs. He gave them a table, and then searched for food for them to share, finding a giant toy carrot, which he placed on the table. As he settled the first little boy into a chair he smiled and said, "that's me."

I knew that his initial approach to other children in his classroom, when he wanted to make contact, was to hit them. In this play he seemed to be actively thinking about a new way to be with others. He became visibly more relaxed—smiling and humming. For me, this indication of another way of being with others was remarkable. It was made more remarkable in that we were together in India, where I was part of the teaching team for a course in therapies and expressive approaches for supporting autism.[1] Our communication through play had reached across cultures, bringing a sense of new possibilities for this small boy with autism.

In both of these sessions, connecting with the child and carefully observing helped me to learn more about their worlds: both the worlds they had created in the sand, and the world of peers and family that they inhabit.

When adults are open to learning from children, they support learning from their experiences, their play, and their art images. First therapists must help children to feel comfortable, finding their way with materials and with ways of playing that may be new to them, whether they dive into the process or wade in slowly.

To create comfort for autistic children and adolescents therapists can start with their interests and preferences. Therapists can create space for them to share what they know and care about. One child spontaneously reflected on the beginning of his therapy, all the while busily pulling out an array of the fidgets that I keep in a basket on my art table, and finding his favorites. I noticed that he had chosen the same ones that he had chosen when we first met. He nodded knowingly. He agreed that playing with the magnets, the prisms, and the stress balls had helped him to feel comfortable in a new place, before he felt ready to do anything else. "Now," he said, "I love to come here!" To create this level of comfort for children, so that they feel comfortable dealing with the challenges that have brought them to therapy, takes a careful balance between following the child's lead and providing structure and support. Following the child's lead enables adults to understand the child's perception of the world more clearly. Offering more structure or direction scaffolds new learning and supports the growth of new abilities in coping and communication.

An integrative approach to therapy allows for dynamic movement between art and play. A flexible, responsive, and individualized way of working enables a broad perspective on what creates change. Art and play allow children to depict emotions and ideas in their own way. These expressive and creative processes allow children to share their stories, even without words. And the therapeutic and expressive languages of art and play provide a multisensory and child-centered way of working with children, one that follows the child's lead but also provides needed supports to encourage the growth of self-regulation and communication.

We connect the mind, brain, and senses through making art and moving through the dynamic process of play. Repetitive play or imagery can shift, as chaos becomes order, and aggression becomes nurturing. Wrestlers molded in clay or played with in the sand can also inhabit the doll's house, tucking children into bed with lovingly decorated blankets of soft felt. Children are able to experience themselves in a new way and patiently work through their frustrations and fears, allowing them to move more freely into new experiences. And children and adolescents alike can recognize new strengths, as they realize the power of an image they have created to capture their feelings or ideas.

For a young adolescent who arrived in my office in a self-described "bad mood," with head down and hood up, the process of creating helped to create movement and perspective after a long and trying day. He began, as did the young child previously described, with poking through my basket of fidgets.

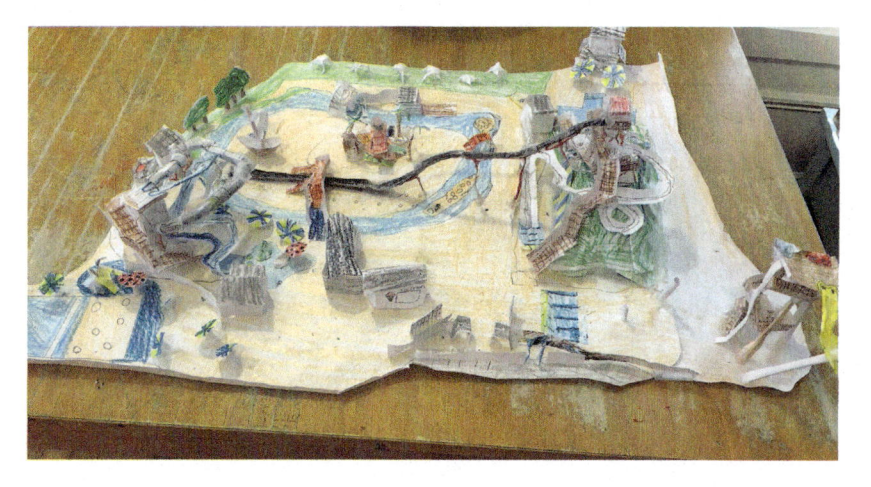

Figure 15.3 Favorite things depicted in a paper world: nature and an amusement park.

Engaging the senses can help build the comfort to create and communicate, no matter how old children are. He then chose some faces for my robot toy, one calm, and one angry, stacking them one on top of the other, and noting, "He's mad AND he's okay." We both realized that he had made the robot look a bit like "Mr. Good/Bad," a figure that he had drawn in an earlier session, and whom he described as feeling "more than one way." His ability to communicate about how confusing mixed feelings can be was impressive. He acknowledged that he too sometimes felt more than one way, particularly when a part of his day may have gone badly, dimming the pleasure of all the things that he had enjoyed and darkening his mood. As we played and talked, I suggested that we try using some clay together, "since we can move the clay, and change it, even squash it or slam it on the table if we feel like it." We both took a hand-sized ball of clay and began to walk around the room together, with a stop to try out smashing the clay on the table. With a growing smile, this boy sat down to transform his clay, patiently working it into a solid ball, then smoothing and shaping and joining his clay into a strongly standing figure. I encouraged him to give this figure a name. With a smile he declared, "He's Mr. Curie." I must have looked puzzled, since he explained, "He's curious about everything." For this boy who was struggling with joining in activities with peers, and persistently asserting that the best choice of what to do might be "nothing," this was an important revelation. Engaging his curiosity, his interests, and his strengths proved to be a path to new, and pleasurable, experiences for him.

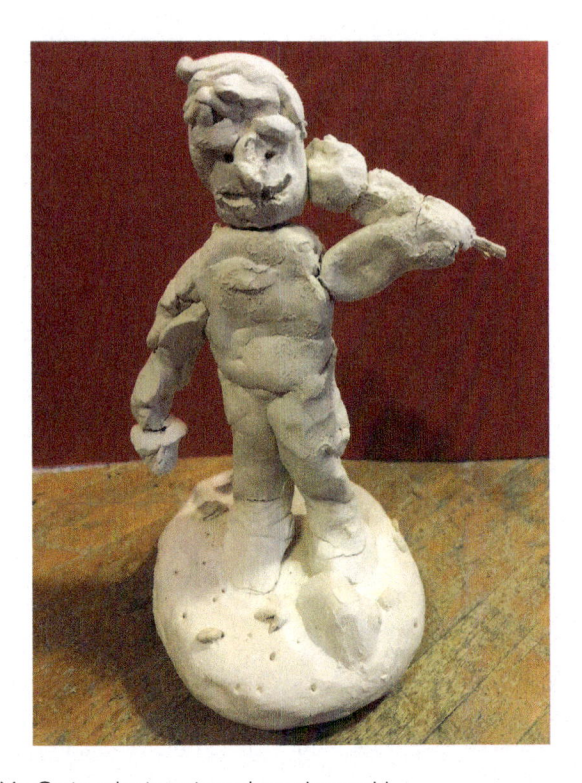

Figure 15.4 Mr. Curie, who is curious about the world.

The potential of art for communication, for calming, and for the expression of feelings "can be a tool to enter a child's world" (R. Mustafa Moury, personal communication, January 14, 2019) one mother realized, as she discussed her autistic child's art with me. This possibility exists at any level of art making, with or without the presence of words to describe what has taken place and what has been created. As she explained, "changing our views" of what it means to make art makes it possible to share creative experiences and "treat our children with joy" (personal communication, January 14, 2019). Through their exploration of color, movement, and the senses, children are being expressive. Through the making and placement of images, or of figures for play, children are being intentional. And when children reflect on what they have created, they share their ideas and feelings. One young child not only added animals he loved to the sand tray, he explored how these creatures were feeling. He suggested to me: "Look at his face! He feels good." When therapists, parents, and teachers respect this process of play, creation, and imagination, then communication and relationships are strengthened and a stronger image of the child will emerge.

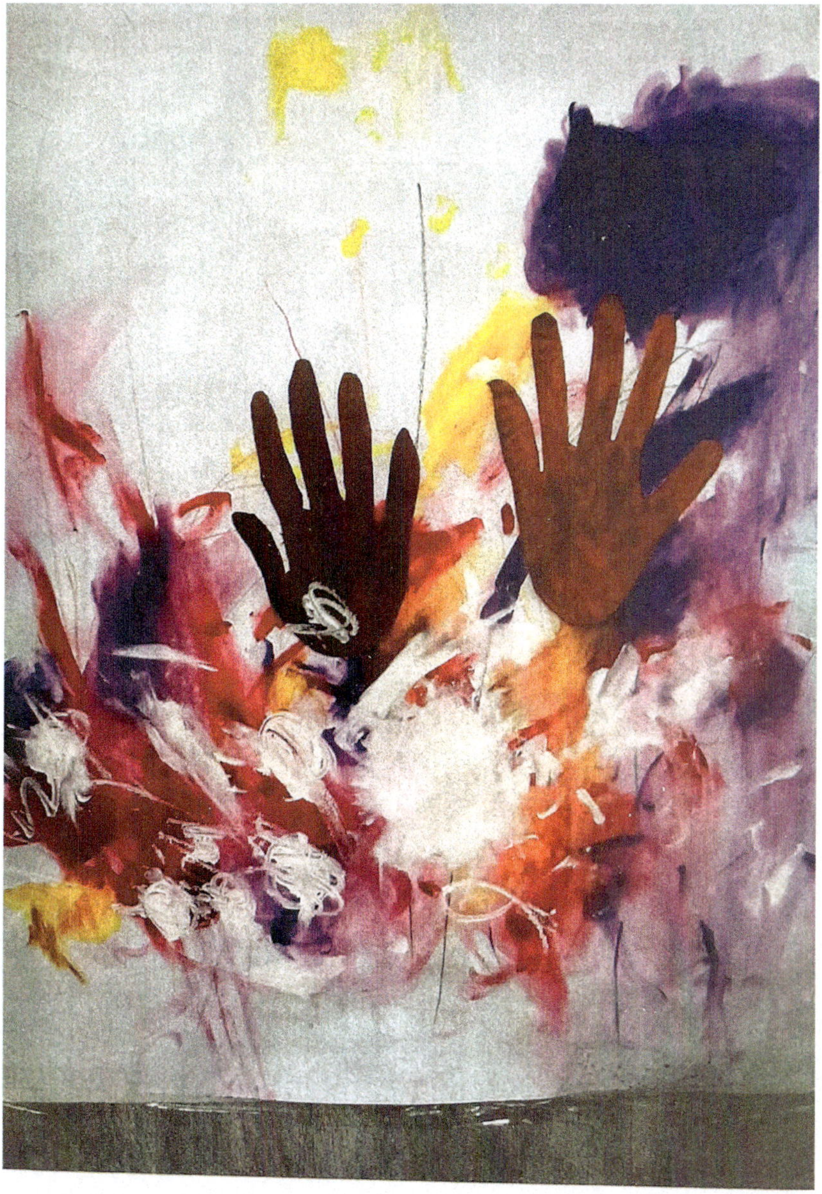

Conclusion 177

Figure 15.5 A child's hands appear in the energetic space of her painting. Used by permission of Rezwana Mustafa.

Note

1 This sand tray was created with a child in the practicum demonstration for a course titled *Autism: Traditional Therapies and Expressive Arts Approaches*. November 2018, Delhi, India.

References

American Psychiatric Association. (1980). *Diagnostic and statistical manual of mental disorders* (3rd ed.). American Psychiatric Publishing.

American Psychiatric Association. (1994). *Diagnostic and statistical manual of mental disorders* (4th ed.). American Psychiatric Publishing.

American Psychiatric Association. (2013). *Diagnostic and statistical manual of mental disorders* (5th ed.). American Psychiatric Publishing.

Ariel, C., & Naseef, R. (2005). *Voices from the spectrum: Parents, grandparents, siblings, people with autism, and professionals share their wisdom*. Jessica Kingsley Publishers.

Ashton, D. (Ed.). (1988). *Picasso on art*. DaCapo.

Askham, A. V. (2020, July 3). Sensory networks overly connected early in autism. *Spectrum*. www.spectrumnews.org/news/sensory-networks-overconnected-early-in-autism/?utm_source=Spectrum+Newsletters&utm_campaign=30516b718f-EMAIL_CAMPAIGN_2020_07_02_01_47&utm_medium=email&utm_term=0_529db1161f-30516b718f-168619701

Athanasiou, F., & Karkou, V. (2017). Establishing relationships with children with autism spectrum disorders through dance movement psychotherapy. In S. Daniel & C. Trevarthen (Eds.), *Rhythms of relating in children's therapies: Connecting creatively with vulnerable children* (pp. 272–292). Jessica Kingsley Publishers.

Attwood, T. (1997). *The complete guide to Asperger's syndrome*. Jessica Kingsley Publishers.

Attwood, T. (2000). In the spotlight: Tony and Temple face to face. *Current Topics in Psychology*. www.fenichel.com/Temple-Tony.html

Attwood, T. (2006). Asperger's syndrome and problems related to stress. In G. Baron, J. Groden, G. Groden, & G. Lipsitt (Eds.), *Stress and coping in autism* (pp. 351–371). Oxford University Press.

Badenoch, B. (2008). *Being a brain-wise therapist: A practical guide to interpersonal neurobiology*. W. W. Norton and Company.

Badenoch, B., & Bogdan, N. (2012). Safety and connection the neurobiology of play. In L. Gallo-Lopez & L. Rubin (Eds.), *Play-based interventions for children and adolescents with autism spectrum disorders* (pp. 3–18). Routledge.

Baron, G., Groden, J., Groden, G., & Lipsitt, L. (Eds.). (2006). *Stress and coping in autism*. Oxford University Press.

Barron-Cohen, S., & Wheelwright, S. (2004). The empathy quotient: An investigation of adults with Asperger Syndrome or high functioning autism, and sex differences. *Journal of Autism and Developmental Disorders, 34*(2), 163–175.

Bauman, M. L. (2015). Foreword to the new edition. In S. M. Edleson (Ed.), *Infantile autism: The syndrome and its implications for a neural theory of behavior by Bernard Rimland, Ph.D.* (pp. 13–15). Jessica Kingsley Publishers.

Berger, D. (2002). *Music therapy, sensory integration, and the autistic child*. Jessica Kingsley Publishers.

Bogdashina, O. (2016). Sensory perceptual issues in autism and Asperger syndrome. In *Different sensory experiences-different perceptual worlds*. Jessica Kingsley Publishers.

Bolte, S. (2020, June 5). *Pluralistic view of autism using the ICF* [Keynote]. INSAR Institute 2020: Developmental Stages of Autism Through a Research Lens.

Bousted, G. (2015, March 11). Debating the merits of "autism" as a diagnostic category. *Spectrum.* www.spectrumnews.org/opinion/cross-talk/cross-talk-debating-the-merits-of-autism-as-a-diagnostic-category/

Bromfield, R. (2010). *Doing therapy with children and adolescents with Asperger's syndrome*. John Wiley and Sons.

Brown, L. (2011). Autism FAQ. *Autistic Hoya.* www.autistichoya.com/p/introduction-to-autism-faqs-of-autism.html

Brown, L. (2019, July 21). Identity-first language. *Autistic Self Advocacy Network.* https://autisticadvocacy.org/about-asan/identity-first-language

Brown, S. (2010). *Play: How it shapes the brain, opens the imagination, and invigorates the soul*. Avery.

Cane, F. (1983). *The artist in each of us*. Art Therapy Publications.

CDC Autism and Developmental Disabilities Monitoring Network. (2018). *Community report from the Autism and Developmental Disabilities Monitoring (ADDM) Network: A snapshot of Autism Spectrum Disorder among 8-year-old children in multiple communities across the United States in 2014*. CDC. www.cdc.gov/ncbddd/autism/addm-community-report/documents/addm-community-report-2018-h.pdf

Chapman, L. (2014). *Neurobiologically informed trauma therapy with children and adolescents: Understanding mechanisms of change*. W. W. Norton and Company.

Chawla, D. (2019, July 3). Large study supports discarding the term 'high-functioning autism'. *Spectrum.* www.spectrumnews.org/news/large-study-supports-discarding-term-high-functioning-autism/

Chilton, G., & Wilkinson, R. (2017). *Positive art therapy theory and practice: Integrating positive psychology with art therapy*. Routledge.

Chown, N., Hughes, L., & Baker-Rogers, J. (2019). What about the other side of double empathy? A response to Alkhaldi, Sheppard and Mitchell's JADD article concerning mind-reading difficulties in autism. *Journal of Autism and Developmental Disorders, 50*(2), 683–684.

Cohen, B., Barnes, M., & Rankin, B. (1995). *Managing traumatic stress through art: Drawing from the center*. Sidran Press.

Collura, L. G. (2012a, March 27). *Leonora speaks: Interview with Jennifer Damian* [Radio broadcast]. Naturally Autistic ANCA.

Collura, L. G. (2012b, April 4). *Leonora speaks: Interview with Jennifer Damian* [Radio broadcast]. Naturally Autistic ANCA.

Collura, L. G. (2012c, May 2). *Leonora speaks: Interview with Jennifer Damian* [Radio broadcast]. Naturally Autistic ANCA.

Courtney, J. (2017). The art of utilizing the metaphorical elements of nature in ecopsychology play therapy. In A. Kopytin & M. Rugh (Eds.), *Environmental expressive therapies: Nature-assisted theory and practice* (pp. 100–122). Routledge.

Cozolino, L. (2010). *The neuroscience of psychotherapy.* W. W. Norton and Company.

Crain, W. (2005). *Theories of development.* Prentice Hall.

Crenshaw, D. (2011, November 5). Fawns in Gorilla Suits. *New England Play Therapy Conference,* Natick, MA.

Csikszentmihalyi, M. (2008). *Flow: The psychology of optimal experience.* Harper Perennial Modern Classics.

Daniel, S., & Trevarthen, C. (2017). Introduction: Rhythm from the beginning. In S. Daniel & C. Trevarthen (Eds.), *Rhythms of relating in children's therapies: Connecting creatively with vulnerable children* (pp. 9–11). Jessica Kingsley Publishers.

Dannecker, K. (2017). Edith Kramer's third hand: Intervention in art therapy. In L. Gerity & S. Annand (Eds.), *The legacy of Edith Kramer: A multifaceted view* (pp. 141–147). Routledge.

Darewych, O. (2018). Digital devices as creative expressive tools for adults with autism. In C. Malchiodi (Ed.), *Art therapy and digital technology* (pp. 317–332). Jessica Kingsley Publishers.

Davis, J. (2017). Drawing nature. In A. Kopytin & M. Rugh (Eds.), *Environmental expressive therapies: Nature-assisted theory and practice* (pp. 63–78). Routledge.

De Domenico, G. (2000). *Comprehensive guide to the use of sand tray in psychotherapy and transformational settings.* Vision Quest Images.

Deweert, S. (2013, May 27). Funding agency shifts focus away from diagnostic groups. *Spectrum.* www.spectrumnews.org/news/funding-agency-shifts-focus-away-from-diagnostic-groups/

Dolphin, M., Byer, A., Goldsmith, A., & Jones, R. (2014). *Psychodynamic art therapy practice with people on the autistic spectrum.* Routledge.

Elbrecht, C. (2012). *Trauma healing at the clay field: A sensorimotor art therapy approach.* Jessica Kingsley Publishers.

Elbrecht, C. (2018). *Healing trauma with guided drawing: A sensorimotor art therapy approach to bilateral body mapping.* North Atlantic Books.

Elkis-Abuhoff, D. (2009). Art therapy and adolescents with Asperger's Syndrome. In S. Brooke (Ed.), *The use of creative therapies with autism spectrum disorders* (pp. 19–42). Charles C. Thomas.

Evans, K., & Dubowski, J. (2001). *Art therapy with children on the autistic spectrum: Beyond words.* Jessica Kingsley.

Fox, L. (1998). Lost in space: The relevance of art therapy with clients who have autism or autistic features. In M. Rees (Ed.), *Drawing on difference: Art therapy with people who have learning difficulties* (pp. 73–91). Routledge.

Franklin, M. (2017). *Art as contemplative practice: Expressive pathways to the self.* SUNY Press.

Furfaro, H. (2017, November 20). Race, class contribute to disparities in autism diagnoses. *Spectrum.* www.spectrumnews.org/news/race-class-contribute-disparities-autism-diagnoses/

Gabriels, R. L. (2003). Art therapy with children who have autism and their families. In C. Malchiodi (Ed.), *Handbook of art therapy* (pp. 193–206). The Guilford Press.

Gallese, V. (2009). Mirror neurons, embodied simulation, and the neural basis of social identification. *Psychoanalytic Dialogues*, *19*, 519–536. http://old.unipr.it/arpa/mirror/pubs/pdffiles/Gallese/Gallese%20PD%202009a.pdf

Gandini, L., Hill, L., Cadwell, L., & Schwall, C. (2005). *In the spirit of the studio: Learning from the atelier of Reggio Emilia*. Teachers College Press.

Gandini, L., & Kaminsky, J. (2005). The construction of the educational project. In C. Rinaldi (Ed.), *In dialogue with Reggio Emilia: Listening, researching, and learning* (pp. 121–136). Routledge.

Gaskill, R., & Perry, D. (2014). The neurobiological power of play: Using the neurosequential model of therapeutics to guide play in the healing process. In C. Malchiodi & D. Crenshaw (Eds.), *Creative arts and play therapy for attachment problems* (pp. 178–194). The Guilford Press.

Gerity, L., & Annand, S. (Eds.). (2017). *The legacy of Edith Kramer: A multifaceted view*. Routledge.

Gil, E., Konrath, E., Shaw, J., Goldin, M., & McTaggart Bryan, H. (2014). Integrative approach to play therapy. In D. Crenshaw & A. Stewart (Eds.), *Play therapy: A comprehensive guide to theory and practice* (pp. 99–113). The Guilford Press.

Goebl-Parker, S., & Richardson, J. (2011). Inspiring our pedagogical imagination: Education through relationships, materials, and images. *Journal of Pedagogy, Pluralism, and Practice*, *4*(3), 71–87. https://digitalcommons.lesley.edu/cgi/viewcontent.cgi?article=1139&context=jppp

Goldberg, L. (2013). *Yoga therapy for children with autism and special needs*. W. W. Norton and Company.

Goucher, C. (2012). Art therapy: Connecting and communicating. In L. Gallo-Lopez & L. Rubin (Eds.), *Play-based interventions for children and adolescents with autism spectrum disorders* (pp. 295–316). Routledge.

Grandin, T. (1996). *Emergence: Labelled autistic*. Warner Books.

Grandin, T. (2006a). *Thinking in pictures: My life with autism*. Vintage.

Grandin, T. (2006b, June). *VSA keynote presentation*. Bold Steps, Washington, DC.

Grandin, T. (2015, July 11). The autistic brain [Masterclass]. *46th annual conference of the American Art Therapy Association*, Minneapolis.

Grandin, T. (2017, October 4). *An evening with Temple Grandin*. University of Massachusetts.

Grandin, T., & Moore, D. (2016). *The loving push: How parents and professionals can help spectrum kids become successful adults*. Future Horizons.

Grandin, T., & Panek, R. (2013). *The autistic brain: Helping different kinds of minds succeed*. Mariner Books.

Grandin, T., & Scariano, M. (2005). *Emergence: Labelled autistic*. Grand Central Publishing.

Grant, R. J. (2017a). *AutPlay therapy for children and adolescents on the autism spectrum: A behavioral play-based approach* (3rd ed.). Routledge/Taylor & Francis Group.

Grant, R. J. (2017b, August 27). *Using art and play in play therapy with children diagnosed with Autism Spectrum Disorders*. Online Play Therapy Summit.

Gray, C. (2002). Welcome to the Jenison Autism Journal: The SCERTS model. *Jenison Autism Journal*, *14*(4).

Green, E. (2012). The Narcissus myth, resplendent reflections, and self-healing: A Jungian perspective on counseling a child with Asperger's Syndrome. In L. Gallo-Lopez &

L. Rubin (Eds.), *Play-based interventions for children and adolescents with autism spectrum disorders*. Routledge.

Greenspan, S. (1996). *The growth of the mind*. Addison Wesley.

Greenspan, S. (2012). Listen to Dr. Greenspan. *The Greenspan Floortime Approach*. www.stanleygreenspan.com/blog

Greenspan, S., & Shanker, S. (2004). *The first idea: How symbols, language, and intelligence evolved from our primate ancestors to modern humans*. Da Capo Press.

Greenspan, S., & Wieder, S. (1998). *The child with special needs*. Perseus Books.

Greenspan, S., & Wieder, S. (2009). *Engaging autism: Using the Floortime approach to help children relate, communicate, and think*. Da Capo Press.

Guest, J. D., & Ohrt, J. H. (2018). Utilizing child-centered play therapy with children diagnosed with autism spectrum disorder and endured trauma: A case example. *International Journal of Play Therapy, 27*(3), 157–165. https://doi.org/10.1037/pla0000074

Happe, F. (2011, March 29). Why fold Asperger syndrome into autism spectrum disorder in the DSM-5? *Spectrum*. www.spectrumnews.org/opinion/viewpoint/why-fold-asperger-syndrome-into-autism-spectrum-disorder-in-the-dsm-5/

Hass-Cohen, N., & Findlay, J. (2015). *Art therapy and the neuroscience of relationships, creativity, and resiliency*. W.W. Norton and Company.

Henley, D. (1992). *Exceptional children exceptional art: Teaching art to children with special needs*. Davis Publications.

Henley, D. (2002). *Clayworks in art therapy: Plying the sacred circle*. Jessica Kingsley Publishers.

Henley, D. (2018). *Creative response activities for children on the spectrum: A therapeutic and educational memoir*. Routledge.

Herbert, M. (2012). *The autism revolution*. Ballantine Books.

Hillman, H. (2018). Child-centered play therapy as an intervention for children with autism: A literature review. *International Journal of Play Therapy, 27*(4), 198–204. https://doi.org/10.1037/pla0000083

Hinz, L. (2009). *Expressive therapies continuum: A framework for using art in therapy*. Routledge.

Hosseini, D. (2012). *The art of autism: Shifting perceptions*. The Art of Autism.

Hull, K. (2014). Play therapy with children on the autism spectrum. In D. Crenshaw & A. Stewart (Eds.), *Play therapy: A comprehensive guide to theory and practice* (pp. 400–414). The Guilford Press.

ICF. (2017). ICF core set for Autism Spectrum Disorder (ASD). *ICF Research Branch*. www.icf-research-branch.org/icf-core-sets-projects2/other-health-conditions/icf-core-set-for-autism-spectrum

Interdisciplinary Council on Developmental and Learning Disorders (Organization). (2000). *Clinical practice guidelines: Redefining the standards of care for infants, children, and families with special needs*. Zero to Three Press.

Jaswal, V., & Akhtar, N. (2018, June 19). *Being vs. appearing socially uninterested: Challenging assumptions about social motivation in autism*. Cambridge University Press. www.cambridge.org/core/journals/behavioral-and-brain-sciences/article/abs/being-versus-appearing-socially-uninterested-challenging-assumptions-about-social-motivation-in-autism/4E75B5E49CC0061E65A4D78552482AF9

Josefi, O., & Ryan, V. (2004). Non-directive play therapy for young children with autism: A case study. *Clinical Child Psychology and Psychiatry, 9*(4), 533–551. https://doi.org/10.1177/1359104504046158

Junge, M. B. (2007). The art therapist as social activist: Reflections on a life. In F. Kaplan (Ed.), *Art therapy and social action* (pp. 40–58). Jessica Kingsley Publishers.
Kagin, S., & Lusebrink, V. (1978). The expressive therapies continuum. *Art Psychotherapy, 5*, 171–180.
Kanner, L. (1943). Autistic disturbances of affective contact. *Nervous child, 2*, 217–250.
Kapitan, L. (2013). Art therapy's sweet spot between art, anxiety, and the flow experience. *Art Therapy: Journal of the American Art Therapy Association, 30*(2), 54–55.
Kaplan, F. (Ed.). (2007). *Art therapy and social action: Treating the world's wounds*. Jessica Kingsley Publishers.
Kaplan, F. (2016). Social action art therapy. In D. Gussak & M. Rosal (Eds.), *The Wiley handbook of art therapy* (pp. 787–793). John Wiley and Sons.
Kaplan, F. (2018, June 10). Art therapists for human rights Facebook page. *Art Therapists for Human Rights*. www.facebook.com/AT4HR/
Karpov, Y. (2005). *The neo-Vygotskian approach to child development*. Cambridge University Press.
Kaufman, S. B. (2012, April 9). Conversation with prodigious savant Daniel Tammet. *The Creativity Post*. www.creativitypost.com/conversations/conversation_with_daniel_tammet
Kellman, J. (2001). *Autism, art and children: The stories we draw*. Bergin and Garvey.
Kestly, T. (2014). *The interpersonal neurobiology of play: Brain building interventions for emotional well-being*. Norton.
Khalsa, S. (1998). *Fly like a butterfly: Yoga for children*. Sterling.
Khalsa, S. (2016). *The yoga way to radiance: How to follow your inner guidance and nurture children to do the same*. Llewellyn Publications.
Kim, J. A., Szatmari, P., Bryson, S. E., Streiner, D. L., & Wilson, F. J. (2000). The prevalence of anxiety and mood problems among children with autism and Asperger syndrome. *Autism, 4*(2), 117–132. https://doi.org/10.1177/1362361300004002002
King, J. (2016). Art therapy: A brain-based profession. In D. Gussak & M. Rosal (Eds.), *The Wiley handbook of art therapy* (pp. 77–89). John Wiley and Sons.
Kopytin, A., & Rugh, M. (Eds.). (2017). *Environmental expressive therapies: Nature-assisted theory and practice*. Routledge.
Kossak, M. (2015). *Attunement in expressive arts therapy: Toward an understanding of embodied empathy*. Charles C. Thomas.
Kramer, E. (1979). *Childhood and art therapy: Notes on theory and application*. Schocken Books.
Kramer, E. (2000). *Art as therapy: Collected papers*. Jessica Kingsley Publishers.
Kranowitz, C. (2006). *The out of sync child: Recognizing and coping with sensory processing disorder*. Tarcher Perigree.
Kranowitz, C. (2018, March 24). The out of sync child [Keynote Presentation]. *Parenting matters conference*, Bradley Hospital, Barrington, RI.
Landolf, H. (2015). Appendix V: My brother, Mark Rimland. In S. M. Edelson (Ed.), *Infantile autism: The syndrome and its implications for a neural theory of behavior by Bernard Rimland, Ph. D.* (pp. 306–311). Jessica Kingsley Publishers.
Lara, J. (2016). *Autism movement therapy method: Waking up the brain*. Jessica Kingsley Publishers.
Lara, J., & Bowers, K. (2013, September/October). Expressive arts: Learning, growing, and expressing. *Autism Asperger's Digest*. http://autismdigest.com/expressive-arts-learning-growing-and-expressing

Lara, J., & Richardson, J. (2019). Energy and nature in the arts and play: Supporting autism. In *Natures et cultures en arts-Therapies: Revue annuelle de la Federation Francaise des Art-Therapeutes*. Federation Francaise des Art-Therapeutes.

Levine, K., & Chedd, N. (2007). *Replays: Using play to enhance emotional and behavioral development for children with autism spectrum disorders*. Jessica Kingsley Publishers.

Liebmann, M. (2004). *Art therapy for groups: A handbook of themes and exercises*. Routledge.

Lord, C. (2020, June 11). *Working with autistic individuals across the lifespan: Current perspectives* [Conference Presentation]. INSAR Institute Research Conference.

Lovecky, D. (2006). *Different minds: Gifted children with AD/HD, Asperger syndrome, and other learning deficits*. Jessica Kingsley Publishers.

Lowenfeld, V. (1975). *Creative and mental growth*. Macmillan.

Lusebrink, V. (1990). *Imagery and visual expression in therapy*. Plenum Press.

Lusebrink, V. (2016). Expressive therapies continuum. In D. Gussak & M. Rosal (Eds.), *The Wiley handbook of art therapy* (pp. 57–67). John Wiley and Sons.

Macari, S., Chen, X., Brunissen, L., Yhang, E., Brennan-Wydra, E., Vernetti, A., Volkmar, F., Chang, J., & Chawarska, K. (2021). Puppets facilitate attention to social cues in children with ASD. *Autism Research*, 1–11. https://doi.org/10.1002/aur.2552

Malchiodi, C. (2003). Art therapy and the brain. In C. Malchiodi (Ed.), *Handbook of art therapy* (pp. 16–24). The Guilford Press.

Malchiodi, C. (2010, October 31). Cool art therapy intervention #1: The art therapist's third hand. *Psychology Today*. www.psychologytoday.com/us/blog/arts-and-health/201010/cool-art-therapy-intervention-1-the-art-therapist-s-third-hand

Malchiodi, C. (Ed.). (2011). *Handbook of creative arts therapy*. The Guilford Press.

Malchiodi, C. (2020). *Trauma and expressive arts therapy: Brain, body and imagination in the healing process*. The Guilford Press.

Malchiodi, C., & Crenshaw, D. (2014). *Creative arts and play therapy for attachment problems*. The Guilford Press.

Malchiodi, C., & Crenshaw, D. (2017). *What to do when children clam up in psychotherapy: Interventions to facilitate communication*. The Guilford Press.

Martin, N. (2009). *Art as an early intervention tool for children with autism*. Jessica Kingsley Publishers.

Mastrangelo, S. (2009). Harnessing the power of play: Opportunities for children with autism spectrum disorders. *TEACHING Exceptional Children*, *41*, 34–44.

McCarthy, D. (2007). *If you turned into a monster*. Jessica Kingsley Publishers.

McGarry, L. M., & Russo, F. A. (2011). Mirroring in dance/movement therapy: Potential mechanisms behind empathy enhancement. *The Arts in Psychotherapy*, *38*(3), 178–184.

McNiff, S. (1995). Keeping the studio. *Art Therapy: The Journal of the American Art Therapy Association*, *12*(3), 179–183. https://doi.org/10.1016/j.aip.2011.04.005

McNiff, S. (1998). *Trust the process: An artist's guide to letting go*. Shambhala Publications.

McNiff, S. (2011, September 21). Arts therapies and the intelligence of feeling [Keynote Address]. *European creative arts therapies conference*. Lucca, Italy.

McNiff, S. (2015). *Imagination in action: Secrets for unleashing creative expression*. Shambhala Publications.

McNiff, S. (2017). Forward: Artistic expression as a force of nature. In A. Kopytin & M. Rugh (Eds.), *Environmental expressive therapies: Nature-assisted theory and practice* (pp. ix–xii). Routledge.

Miller, A., & Eller-Miller, E. (1989). *From ritual to repertoire: A cognitive-developmental systems approach with behavior-disordered children*. John Wiley and Sons.

Miller, E. (2008). *Autism through art: The girl who spoke with pictures*. Jessica Kingsley Publishers.

Miller, L., Goodwin, M., & Sullivan, J. (2015). Rimland's contributions: The role of sensory processing challenges in autism spectrum disorders. In E. Edelson (Ed.), *Infantile autism: The syndrome and its' implications for a neural theory of behavior* (pp. 149–155). Jessica Kingsley Publishers.

Mills, J. (2014). Storyplay: A narrative play therapy approach. In D. Crenshaw & A. Stewart (Eds.), *Play therapy: A comprehensive guide to theory and practice*. The Guilford Press.

Milton, D. (2012). On the ontological status of autism: The double empathy problem. *Disability and Society, 27*, 883–887.

Mitchell, P. (2016). *Mindreading as a transactional process: Insights from autism*. Routledge.

Moat, D. (2013). *Integrative psychotherapeutic approaches to autism spectrum conditions*. Jessica Kingsley Publishers.

Moon, B. (2008). *Introduction to art therapy: Faith in the process*. Charles C. Thomas.

Moon, C. (2010). *Materials and media in art therapy: Critical understandings of diverse artistic vocabularies*. Routledge.

Mullin, J. (2015). *Drawing autism*. Akashic Books.

Mundy, P. (2020, June 3). *Developmental stages of autism through a research lens* [Keynote Presentation]. INSAR.

Muzikar, D. (2016, October 5). An interview with Steve Silberman, author of Neurotribes. *The Art of Autism*. https://the-art-of-autism.com/an-interview-with-steve-silberman-author-of-neurotribes/

Myers, M. (2009). Reaching through the silence: Play therapy in the treatment of children with autism. In S. Brooke (Ed.), *The use of the creative therapies with autism spectrum disorders* (pp. 123–139). Charles C. Thomas.

Nader-Grosbois, N., & Mazzone, S. (2014). Emotion regulation, personality and social adjustment in children with autism spectrum disorders. *Psychology, 5*, 1750–1767. https://doi.org/10.4236/psych.2014.515182

Nemetz, L. D. (2006). Moving with meaning: The historical progression of dance/movement therapy. In S. L. Brooke (Ed.), *Creative arts therapies manual: A guide to the history, theoretical approaches, assessment, and work with special populations of art, play, dance, music, drama, and poetry therapies* (pp. 95–108). Charles C. Thomas.

Opar, A. (2019, April 24). In search of truce in the autism wars. *Spectrum*. www.spectrumnews.org/features/deep-dive/search-truce-autism-wars/

Orbach, N. (2020). *The good enough studio: Art therapy through the prism of space, matter, and action*. Nona Orbach.

Osborne, N. (2017). Love, rhythm, and chronobiology. In S. Daniel & C. Trevarthen (Eds.), *Rhythms of telating in children's therapies: Connecting creatively with vulnerable children* (pp. 14–27). Jessica Kingsley Publishers.

Park, C. (2001). *Exiting nirvana: A daughter's life with autism*. Little Brown and Company.

Penfold, L. (2019, March 12). Vygotsky on collective creativity. *Art. Play. Children. Learning*. www.louisapenfold.com/collective-creativity-vygotsky/

Pliske, M., & Balboa, L. (2019). *Integrating yoga and play therapy: The mind-body approach for healing adverse childhood experiences*. Jessica Kingsley Publishers.

Porges, S. (2011). *The polyvagal theory*. W. W. Norton and Company.

Prizant, B. (2015). *Uniquely human: A different way of seeing autism*. Simon and Schuster.

Prizant, B., Wetherby, A., Rubin, E., Laurent, A., & Rydell, P. (2006). *The SCERTS model: A comprehensive educational approach for children with autism spectrum disorders*. Paul H. Brookes Publishing.

Prizant, B., Wetherby, A., & Rydell, P. (2000). Communication intervention issues for children with autism spectrum disorders. In A. Wetherby & B. Prizant (Eds.), *Autism spectrum disorders: A transactional developmental perspective, volume 9* (pp. 193–224). Paul H. Brookes.

Proulx, L. (2002). *Strengthening emotional ties through parent-child-dyad art therapy*. Jessica Kingsley Publishers.

Ray, D., Sullivan, J., & Carllson, S. (2012). Relational intervention: Child-centered play therapy with children on the autism spectrum. In L. Gallo-Lopez & L. Rubin (Eds.), *Play-based interventions for children and adolescents with autism spectrum disorders* (pp. 159–176). Routledge.

Regensburg, E. (2016, February 16). Why children on the spectrum benefit from art therapy as a required service. *The Art of Autism*. https://the-art-of-autism.com/why-children-on-the-spectrum-benefit-from-art-therapy-as-a-required-service/

Reggio Children (Organization). (1987). *The hundred languages of children*. Reggio Children.

Reggio Children (Organization). (2015). *International study group on children with special rights*, Emilia, Italy.

Rhyne, J. (1984). *The gestalt art experience: Creative process and expressive therapy*. Magnolia Street Publishers.

Richardson, J. (2009). Creating a safe space for adolescents on the autism spectrum. In S. Brooke (Ed.), *The use of creative therapies with autism spectrum disorders* (pp. 103–122). Charles C. Thomas.

Richardson, J. (2012). The world of the sandtray and the child on the autism spectrum. In L. Gallo-Lopez & L. Rubin (Eds.), *Play-based interventions for children and adolescents with autism spectrum disorders* (pp. 209–227). Routledge.

Richardson, J. (2016). Art therapy on the autism spectrum: Engaging the mind, brain, and sense. In D. Gussak & M. Rosal (Eds.), *The Wiley handbook of art therapy* (pp. 306–316). John Wiley and Sons.

Richardson, J., Gollub, A., & Wang, C. (2012). Inkdance: Body, mind, and Chinese medicine as sources for art therapy. In D. Kalmanowitz, J. Potash, & S. Chan (Eds.), *Art therapy in Asia: To the bone or wrapped in silk* (pp. 65–77). Jessica Kingsley Publishers.

Riley-Hall, E. (2012). *Parenting girls on the autism spectrum: Overcoming the challenges and celebrating the gifts*. Jessica Kingsley Publishers.

Rinaldi, C. (2007, June 27–29). Teachers, children, and families as co-researchers [Keynote Presentation]. *NAREA conference*, Santa Monica, CA.

Robbins, A., & Sibley, L. (1976). *Creative art therapy*. Brunner/Mazel.
Ross, M. (2011). *Cultivating the arts in education and therapy*. Routledge.
Rubin, J. (2005). *Child art therapy*. John Wiley and Sons.
Schadler, G., & De Domenico, G. (2012). Sandtray-worldplay for people who experience chronic mental illness. *International Journal of Play Therapy, 21*(2), 87–99.
Schuler, A., & Wolfberg, P. (2000). Promoting peer play and socialization: The art of scaffolding. In A. Wetherby & B. Prizant (Eds.), *Autism spectrum disorders a transactional developmental perspective* (pp. 251–278). Paul. H. Brookes.
Schweizer, C., Knorth, E. J., & Spreen, M. (2014). Art therapy with children with autism spectrum disorders: A review of clinical case descriptions on "what works". *The Arts in Psychotherapy, 41*(5), 577–593.
Sharma, S. (2020, August 11). Anshuman Kar, a non-verbal painter with autism, reveals hidden depths of feeling in his art. *Newz Hook*. https://newzhook.com/story/anshuman-kar-non-verbal-painter-autism-autistic-awesome-artist-ashu-action-for-autism-afa-shaloo-sharma-evoluer-solutions-instagram-artists-autistic/
Sheffer, E. (2019). *Asperger's children: The origins of autism in Nazi Vienna*. W.W. Norton and Company.
Shore, S. (2006a). *Beyond the wall: Personal experiences with autism and Asperger syndrome*. Autism Asperger Publishing Company.
Shore, S. (2006b). *Understanding autism for dummies*. John Wiley and Sons.
Shore, S. (2013). *Exploring autism—from the inside out—through movement and music* [Presentation]. Autism Movement Therapy, New York.
Siegel, D. (2012). *The developing mind: How relationships and the brain interact to shape who we are*. The Guilford Press.
Siegel, D., & Bryson, T. (2012). *The whole brain child: Revolutionary strategies to nurture your child's developing mind survive everyday parenting struggles and help your child thrive*. Delacourte Press.
Siegel, D., & Hartzell, M. (2013). *Parenting from the inside out: How a deeper self-understanding can help you raise children who thrive*. Tarcher.
Silberman, S. (2015). *Neurotribes: The legacy of autism and the future of neurodiversity*. Avery.
Silberman, S., & Foye, R. (2020, May 6). Steve Silberman with Raymond Foye (No. 37) [Interview]. In *The New Social Environment*. The Brooklyn Rail. https://brooklynrail.org/events/2020/05/06/steve-silberman-with-raymond-foye/
Stagnitti, K., & Pfeifer, L. I. (2017). Methodological considerations for a directive play therapy approach for children with autism and related disorders. *International Journal of Play Therapy, 26*(3), 160–171. https://doi.org/10.1037/pla0000049
Steele, W., & Malchiodi, C. (2012). *Trauma informed practices with children and adolescents*. Routledge.
Stern, D. (1985). *The interpersonal world of the infant: A view from psychoanalysis and developmental psychology*. Basic Books, Inc.
Swank, J. M., Walker, K. L. A., & Shin, S. M. (2020). Indoor nature-based play therapy: Taking the natural world inside the playroom. *International Journal of Play Therapy, 29*(3), 155–162. https://doi.org/10.1037/pla0000123
Tortora, S. (2006). *The dancing dialogue: Using the communicative power of movement with young children*. Brookes Publishing.

Treffert, D. (2013, April 12). Darold Treffert M. D. talks about myths about autism and savant artists. *The Art of Autism*. https://the-art-of-autism.com/dr-darold-treffert-myths-about-autism/?fbclid=IwAR0t5rwPnYNYj-IAjPVSSs89wGSNDl7BA2uLxoumq4Izeb2KG1CjMqR6bgU

Trevarthen, C. (2017). Health and happiness grow in play. In S. Daniel & C. Trevarthen (Eds.), *Rhythms of relating in children's therapies* (pp. 28–44). Jessica Kingsley Publishers.

University of Western Australia. (2019, June 20). Researchers call for the term 'high functioning autism' to be consigned to history. *Medical Xpress*. https://medicalxpress.com/news/2019-06-term-high-functioning-autism-consigned.html

Van Briessen, F. (1998). *The way of the brush: Painting techniques of China and Japan*. Charles E. Tuttle.

Van Lith, T., Stallings, J., & Harris, C. (2017). Discovering good practice for art therapy with children who have autism spectrum disorder: The results of a small scale survey. *Arts in Psychotherapy, 54*, 78–84.

Vecchi, V. (2010). *Art and creativity in Reggio Emilia: Exploring the role and potential of ateliers in early childhood education*. Routledge.

Vecchi, V., & Giudici, C. (Eds.). (2004). *Children, art, artists: The expressive languages of children, the artistic language of Alberto Burri*. Reggio Children.

Vygotsky, L. (1978). *Mind in society: The development of higher psychological processes*. Harvard University Press.

Wadeson, H. (1987). *The dynamics of art psychotherapy*. John Wiley and Sons.

Walker, N. (2014, March 1). What is autism? *Neurocosmopolitanism*. https://neurocosmopolitanism.com/what-is-autism/

Weinstock, C. (2019, July 31). The deep emotional ties between depression and autism. *Spectrum*. www.spectrumnews.org/features/deep-dive/the-deep-emotional-ties-between-depression-and-autism/

Weiser, J. (1999). *Phototherapy techniques: Exploring the secrets of personal snapshots and family albums* (2nd ed.). PhotoTherapy Centre Press.

Werner, H. (2012). *Comparative psychology of mental development*. Percheron Press.

Wetherby, A. M., & Prizant, B. M. (Eds.). (2000). *Autism spectrum disorders: A transactional developmental perspective*. Paul H. Brookes Publishing.

Wetherby, A. M., Prizant, B. M., & Schuler, A. (2000). Understanding the nature of communication and language impairments. In A. M. Wetherby & B. Prizant (Eds.), *Autism spectrum disorders a transactional developmental perspective* (pp. 109–142). Paul. H. Brookes.

WHO. (2021, June 1). Autism spectrum disorders. *World Health Organization*. www.who.int/news-room/fact-sheets/detail/autism-spectrum-disorders

Wilkerson, L. (2008, November 20). Sidecars follow-up session [Panelist, Plenary Session]. *American Art Therapy Association conference*, Cleveland, OH.

Wing, L. (1997). The history of ideas on autism. Legends, myths, and reality. *Autism: The International Journal of Research and Practice, 1*(1), 13–23.

Wing, L. (2005). Reflections on opening Pandora's box. *Journal of Autism and Developmental Disorders, 35*(2), 197–203. www.researchgate.net/journal/Journal-of-Autism-and-Developmental-Disorders-1573-3432

Winnicott, D. (2005). *Playing and reality* (2nd ed.). Routledge.

Wolfberg, P. (2003). *Play and imagination in children with autism*. Teachers College Press.

Wright, J. (2015, January 2). Questions for Eric London: Alternative diagnoses for autism. *Spectrum*. www.spectrumnews.org/opinion/questions-for-eric-london-alternative-diagnoses-for-autism/

Zeldovich, L. (2018, May 9). Why the definition of autism needs to be refined. *Spectrum*. www.spectrumnews.org/features/deep-dive/definition-autism-needs-refined/

Zero to three (Organization). (2016). *DC:0–5: Diagnostic classification of mental health and developmental disorders of infancy and early childhood*. Zero to Three Press.

Zoja, E. (2011). *Sandplay in vulnerable communities: A Jungian approach*. Routledge.

Index

acceptance 48, 73, 81
adolescents 1, 4–6, 8, 11, 14–15, 17, 21–22, 24–27, 32–33, 36, 46, 53, 55, 70, 73, 81, 86–88, 90, 93–95, 97, 108–111, 115, 117–118, 125–127, 129–135, 137–140, 145–146, 148–150, 154, 159, 171–172, 174
aesthetic choice 146
Akhtar, N. 47, 119
American Psychiatric Association 49, 52
Anderson, J. 169
anger 26, 83, 91, 101, 122, 130–131, 139, 156
animal figures 1, 15, 168–169, 173, 176; and clay 103–104, 106; in integrative approach 70, 73, 77–78, 89; and sand tray 60, 62–64, 66–67
anxiety 5–6, 17–18, 46, 53, 94, 145; in adolescents 129–133, 135, 137; and feelings 40; in integrative approach 78, 82, 84–85, 87; and perfectionism 113, 115
Applied Behavior Analysis protocol 165
artism 21
artists 21, 106, 150, 160–161, 163, 169
art therapy 17, 24, 27, 30, 32, 75, 81, 95–97, 130, 142–143, 145, 148, 151, 158
Asperger's disorder 49–50
Athanasiou, F. 96, 154
attunement 154, 164–165, 167–168
Attwood, T. 46, 112, 121
Autism Movement Therapy (AMT) 4, 14n1, 165–167
Autism Spectrum Disorder (ASD) 45, 47–49, 52, 55, 87, 93
AutPlay Therapy 75

Badenoch, B. 27, 55, 63, 71, 78, 89–90
balance: in body and in brain 86–92; of child-centered and structured approaches 71; of flexibility and structure 81; between following the child's lead and providing direction 75, 174; of mind, body, and senses 159
Balboa, L. 84
Barron-Cohen, S. 47, 51, 117
Bauman, M. L. 52
behaviors: as accepted means of communication 109; challenging behaviors 78, 86; observation of 47; repetitive 53, 62, 87, 130, 154, 156; self-soothing 16, 85, 96, 111; symbolic 16–17, 22–23, 27, 34, 44, 57, 60, 63, 71, 73, 95–96, 100, 144, 155, 158
Berger, D. 16, 123
biological origins of autism 51
bodily experience 46, 123
body (the body in autism) 95
body tracing 155
Bogdan, N. 78
Bogdashina, O. 143–144, 146, 151, 156, 160
Bolte, S. 50
bop bag 78, 110
bottom-up 152
brain 150; balance in 86–92; connectivity 51; horizontal integration in 88–89; imaging 47; left and right, integration between 95; vertical integration in 89
breathing 75, 84–87, 96, 113, 143
Bromfield, R. 55, 73, 130
Brown, L. 45, 49
bubble wrap 13–14, 143
Burri, A. 143

calming act 5, 8, 11, 38, 149, 151, 154, 168, 176; and adolescents 125, 129–130, 132, 135; in integrative approach 83, 85, 89, 91–92; and perfectionism 109–113; and sand tray 59, 62; and trust 95
Cane, F. 86
Canha, J. 21, 132
cardboard 146–147, 169
Cardillo, N. J. 123
Centers for Disease Control (CDC) 48
Challenges (in autism) 4–6, 11, 13, 16, 19, 22, 25–26, 29–30, 37, 46–47, 49–56, 62, 72–73, 76, 85–87, 93–94, 96–97, 101, 104, 110, 113–114, 118, 125–126, 129–130, 132–133, 135, 144–145, 149–151, 164–165, 167, 174
Chapman, L. 91
Chedd, N. 53
child-centered therapy 57, 63, 70–71, 73–74, 81, 174
childhood disintegrative disorder 49
Chilton, G. 131
Chinese art 159
Chown, N. 45
clamming up 19
clay 1, 17, 25, 96, 98–107, 120, 142, 151, 168–169; as frustrating and rewarding material 153–154; grammar of 105; in integrative approach 70, 76–77; language of 89, 105–106; modelling 37–38, 89, 174–175; and perfectionism 109, 112; physical gestures and body language 101–103; polychrome clay 112; polymer clay 98; shaping 8, 149, 172; varieties 101–102; visual language of 100, 106; working with 89–90
closure/satisfaction in activity 101
cognition 52–53, 89, 160
cognitive processing/intervention 31, 36, 51–53, 89, 117–118, 122, 146, 155, 158–159, 167
Cohen, B. 112
Collura, L. G. 163–164, 168–169
colors 8, 12, 14, 48, 176; and adolescents 125, 129–132; autism spectrum and continuum 143–145, 147, 150, 153–154, 161; and clay 104–106; and engagement of children in therapy 15–17, 22, 24–25; in integrative approach 78, 80, 84; and perfectionism 112, 115; and sand tray 59, 69–70; and strong image 28; and trust 94–95, 97–98
comforting/comfort level 4, 7–9, 13, 42, 46, 171, 173–175; in adolescents 126, 129–135, 137–139; and autism spectrum and continuum 142, 148–149, 151, 154–155, 158; and clay 98, 104, 106; and empathy 118–121; engagement of children in therapy 16–17, 19, 22–24; in integrative approach 74–75, 77–78, 80, 84–85, 87–88, 90–92; and perfectionism 108–109, 112–115, 117; and sand tray 62, 64, 66; and strong image of the child 33–34; and trust 93–96
communication 13–16, 33, 57–59, 81, 145, 174; and behavior 109; challenges 51–53; reciprocal communication 19; social communication 4–6, 22–23, 144–145, 172; support for 23–24, 28, 33; symbolic 16–17, 22–23, 27, 34, 44, 57, 60, 63, 71, 73, 95–96, 100, 144, 155, 158
community 4, 29, 31, 33, 78, 118, 160, 163, 169, 171
connections/connecting 27, 41, 55, 87, 94, 108, 110, 118, 121, 129, 135, 153–154, 167, 174; children/adolescents–creations 20, 90, 149, 160; children/adolescents–interests 8, 42, 57, 122; children/adolescents–materials 1, 8, 78, 91, 106, 126; children/adolescents–others 19, 31–34, 46–47, 52, 64, 68, 87, 96, 103–104, 109, 138, 166, 171; children/adolescents–therapists 6, 8, 17, 26, 28–29, 31, 33, 39, 52, 73, 75–76, 78, 126, 139–140, 153, 173; resources for 4, 26, 105, 146, 167; *see also* materials
continuum 6, 50, 53, 142, 150–155, 158–159
coping/coping strategies 5, 82, 104, 109
Courtney, J. 8
Cozolino, L. 46
crayons 8, 78, 111, 115, 131, 147, 152
creative embodiment 95
creative engagement 159
creative experiences 84, 142, 145, 150, 159, 176

creative expression 29, 31, 34, 83, 91, 159
creative process 28–30
creative response 72–73, 129
creative strategies 95, 167
creativity 16, 55, 62, 159–162, 164; and adolescents 129, 132, 140; and engagement of children in therapy 19, 22, 27; in integrative approach 70, 84, 86, 97; and strong image 29, 31–32
Crenshaw, D. 19, 31–32, 63, 86
cushions 19, 22, 84, 87, 111

Damian, J. 163–170
Damian, K. 164–170
dance 9, 15–16, 18, 39, 63, 91, 96, 163–167
Dannecker, K. 24–25
Darewych, O. 149
Davis, J. 129
DC: 0–5 54–55
De Domenico, G. 13, 27, 57, 63, 68, 71
depressed mood 46, 91, 130
depression 5, 46, 53, 91, 94, 115, 129–130, 135
development 21, 23, 33, 44, 47, 51, 57, 105, 118–119, 132, 150, 152–153, 159–160, 163, 168
diagnosis 45–46; ASD and 48–49, 52–53; behavior observation 47; brain imaging 47; Diagnostic Classification of Mental Health and Developmental Disorders of Infancy and Early Childhood 54; DSM III 52; DSM IV 49; DSM V 50; goals of 6, 46; history of 51–56
digital media 147–149
direction, from therapists 11, 24, 75, 82, 101, 129, 133, 174
DIR Floortime (Greenspan) 14n1, 165
disability 45, 50, 94
disorder, autism as 45
doll's house 1, 70, 83, 108, 171, 174
Dolphin, M. 33, 145
double empathy problem 118–119
drawing 1, 4, 6, 8, 168–169, 172; and adolescents 125–127, 129–132, 134–135, 140; and autism spectrum and continuum 144, 148–149, 151, 153–156, 158–159; and clay 104, 108; and empathy 117–118, 120, 123–124; engagement of children in therapy

16–18, 21, 25–26; and feelings 36–37, 39, 41, 43; in integrative approach 70, 78, 90; and perfectionism 110–111, 114–115; and sand tray 57, 68–69; and trust 94, 96
dreams 18, 22, 62, 66
drums 14–15, 19, 22, 36, 40, 80, 116, 164
Dubowski, J. 16, 24, 142, 151
dynamic language, of play 106
dysregulation 37, 71, 78, 85–86, 91, 152

early intervention 48, 55
Elbrecht, C. 101
embodied art therapy approaches 96, 133
EMDR 85
emotional regulation 4, 51, 81, 88, 117, 119–120, 167; challenges in 16, 22, 62, 144; and materials 87; support for 24, 46, 88
emotions 27, 41, 51, 60, 95, 123, 159, 167; awareness of 121, 158, 166; communicating/expressing 32, 36–44, 63, 70, 73, 86, 88, 126–127, 131–132, 155, 161, 167, 174; dealing with 89–90; emotional upsets, impact of 111; evoking 145–146; exploration of 4–5, 104, 109, 126–127, 129–130, 160–161; and sand tray 12, 37; and stress 85
empathy 117; empathetic relationship 55; empathetic understanding 11; empathic body connection 123; as relational and transactional process 119
energy level 8, 24, 46, 95, 151, 153, 159, 166; and clay 100, 105; and adolescents 131, 133, 135, 140
environment 38, 87, 95, 163, 169, 171; created by children 70; exploration of 22, 24, 97; individual's interaction with 47, 50; learning 32; natural 168; and sand tray 57, 60, 63; school 106; social 32, 158; stimuli, sensitivity to 16, 144; and strong image 29–30, 32–33, 35; support from 16, 29, 32–33; therapeutic 1, 8, 23, 28, 33, 108, 115, 119, 145, 165, 168
Evans, K. 16, 24, 142, 151
expanding sphere balls 87, 113
expressive arts 37, 95

expressive languages 15–17, 28, 31–32, 37, 39, 70
expressive therapies continuum 142, 150, 154, 159; cognitive/symbolic level 158–159; creative level 159–162; and development process 150; perceptual/affective level 155–158; sensorimotor-affective level 159; sensory/kinaesthetic level of 150–151, 154–155

facial expressions 89
family sessions 121–122, 154
fear 11, 13, 38, 81, 93, 103, 115, 144–145, 156, 174; and adolescents 126, 130–131, 133–135; and sand tray 66–68
feelings 17, 32, 36–44, 160, 171, 174–176; and adolescents 126–129, 133–135; awareness of 90–91; challenging 118; and clay figures 102, 104, 106; and colors 70–71, 84, 131; of dysregulation 78; exploration of 36, 40, 43, 80, 89–90, 140; expression of 18, 21, 40, 161; identification of 4, 43; in integrative approach 73, 75, 85–86; language of 32, 36–44; of materials 105, 149–150; and paintings 153; and puppets 110; and sand tray 41, 62, 64, 107; timeline of 82; *see also* empathy
fidgets 9, 22, 72, 78, 87, 113, 174
Findlay, J. 89, 95–96, 102–103
fixated interests, connecting with 42–44
flexibility 4, 8, 51, 57, 165, 169, 171–172; and autism spectrum and continuum 143, 149, 154–155, 158; and clay 104; and empathy 121; and engagement of children in therapy 16–17, 24, 27; in integrative approach 70–71, 80–81, 86, 91; and perfectionism 109, 113; and strong image 33, 38–39; and trust 95, 97
flexible approach 36, 74, 110
flexible materials 8, 39, 91, 143, 149, 172
Floortime 165
flow state 130
focus, working with 21–22
focused interests 55, 130
"Follow Me" Approach 75
Foye, Raymond 6
Franklin, M. 123

friends/friendship 7, 26, 68, 110, 159, 166–167, 169, 171–172; and adolescents 125, 127, 132–133, 140–141; and clay 103, 106; in integrative approach 73, 75–77; and strong image 30, 33
frustration 13, 25–26, 48, 57, 82, 100–101, 110–112, 131, 137, 156, 174

Gallese, V. 119
Gaskill, R. 39
gestures 15, 24, 28, 73, 89, 96, 100–101, 112, 131, 143, 147
Gil, E. 71
Goldberg, L. 84, 86, 111
Goucher, C. 121, 145
grammar: of clay 105; of expression 101; of materials 100
Grandin, T. 19, 21, 23, 37, 39, 45, 47, 49, 55, 62, 93, 101, 110, 112, 143, 146, 158
Grant, R. J. 75, 87, 94
Gray, C. 145
Green, E. 62
Greenspan, S. 16, 27, 47, 52, 55, 63, 73, 97, 163–165, 167
Guest, J. D. 86

Happe, F. 47
Hass-Cohen, N. 89, 95–96, 102–103
Henley, D. 16, 23, 26, 36, 72, 82–83, 97, 135, 144, 153
Herbert, M. 46, 51–52, 55, 95, 142
high functioning autism 50
Hinz, L. 143, 151, 154–156, 158
holistic support 4, 23, 29, 46–47, 165
hope, sense of 109
Hosseini, D. 150
Howard, K. 16
Hull, K. 72

identity 21, 45, 49, 69
images 12, 22, 24, 34, 41, 43, 59–60, 63, 68–69, 83, 94, 96, 98, 101, 104–106, 113–114, 120, 123, 125, 129, 132–134, 140, 146, 148, 150–151, 154–156, 158, 163, 169, 172, 174, 176
imagination 1, 11, 33–34, 118, 133, 145, 176
improvisation 102–103, 137, 145
individualized approach 4, 14n1, 30, 33, 46, 50, 55, 144, 164, 174

integration 14n1, 56, 60, 74, 81, 86–91, 95, 142, 152, 164–166
integrative approach 4, 6, 34, 70–92, 105, 142, 153, 165–166, 174
intentions, understanding of 1–4, 8–11, 34, 93
interactive window approach 155
Interdisciplinary Council on Developmental and Learning Disorders (ICDL) 55
interests: building, in children 18–19; connecting with 8, 42, 57, 122; fixated interests 42–44; focused interests 55, 130; natural interests 57–59, 63; sharing of 33; special interests 1, 8, 18–19, 30, 41–44, 47, 53, 81, 120–122; understanding of 1–4, 8–11, 31
International Classification of Functioning (ICF) 50
interpersonal neurobiology 27

Jaswal, V. 47, 119
Junge, M. B. 32

Kagin, S. 146
kaleidescopes 80, 87
Kanner, L. 45, 51
Kapitan, L. 130
Kaplan, F. 32–33
Karkou, V. 96, 154
Kellman, J. 21
Kestly, T. 60, 87, 91, 96
Khalsa, S. 8, 84, 129
Kim, J. A. 46
kinaesthetic 21, 24, 57, 59, 62, 94, 96, 101–102, 105, 112, 118, 123, 140, 142–143, 150–151, 153–155, 158, 160, 166
kinaesthetic empathy 123
kinaesthetic experiences 24, 94, 96, 112, 142, 151
kinaesthetic process 62, 101, 105, 154
kinaesthetic/sensory level 150–151, 154, 158
King, J. 90
Kossak, M. 46, 91
Kramer, E. 24–25, 101, 158
Kranowitz, C. 143

languages: of children 28–29; of clay 89, 105–106; dynamic language of play 106; expressive 15–17, 28, 31–32, 37, 39, 70; of feelings 32, 36–44; nonverbal 15; verbal 15, 39, 62–63, 106; visual 15–16, 30, 100, 106, 158; *see also* communication
Lara, Joanne 4, 74, 88, 91, 166–167, 169
lead of children 75, 78, 174
Levine, K. 53
listening 1, 15–27, 62–64, 103–104, 129, 172; deep listening 27; and feeling 36, 39–40; in integrative approach 77, 83, 85; to the sound of the ocean 85; and strong image 31–33; watchful "listening" 104
"living language, living symbols" 27, 59, 63
London, Eric 50, 53
Lord, C. 49–50
Lovecky, D. 18–19, 121
Lowenfeld, V. 94, 155
Lusebrink, V. 142, 146, 150–151, 159

Macari, S. 73
magnets 72, 174
Malchiodi, C. 19, 27, 31, 37, 63, 84, 86–87, 95–96, 154
mark making 96, 150–151, 155
Martin, N. 100, 145–146, 152, 154–155
materials 1, 14, 36, 87, 109, 113, 144, 146–148; and adolescents 120, 129, 132; for breathing 85; children/adolescents connection with 1, 8, 78, 91, 106, 126; different feelings and different possibilities 149; and emotional regulation 87; and engagement of children in therapy 15, 22, 26; and evocation 145; expressive qualities of 132; feelings of 40–44, 105, 149–150; flexible 8, 39, 91, 143, 149, 172; freedom to change 112; grammar of 100; and matching 152; for movement 40; natural 105–106, 112–113, 132, 135; nature of 146–150; open-ended materials 39, 112, 145, 171; preferences 146–147; psychology of 150; responsive 8, 39, 91, 98, 143, 149, 151; sensory 19, 24, 72, 87, 98, 112, 139–140, 147, 154, 159, 171; and strong image 32–33; traditional art materials 17, 121, 147–148; *see also specific types*
Mazzone, S. 117

McGarry, L. M. 166–167
McNiff, S. 14, 93–94, 100, 145, 159
media 22, 38, 121, 130–131, 146–148, 159
meltdowns 86–87
metaphorical play 94
metaphors 70, 101
microgenetic mobility 160–162
Miller, A. 151, 155
Miller, E. 21
Miller, K. 21
Miller, L. 95, 142
Mills, J. 78
Milton, D. 119
mind 4, 17, 21, 31, 40, 45–46, 49, 68, 81, 86, 95, 101, 117–118, 142, 158–159, 163–164, 167, 169, 174
mirroring 70, 96, 102, 133, 154–155, 166–167
Mitchell, P. 119
Moat, D. 47, 53, 55
"modified, naturalistic, ABA" therapy 165
Moon, B 135, 145
Moon, C. 20, 150
movements 13, 16, 20, 29, 32, 36–37, 53, 174, 176; and adolescents 125, 130–133; Autism Movement Therapy (AMT) 4, 14n1, 165–167; autism spectrum and continuum 142, 145, 150–151, 153–155, 160; of the body 39; and clay figures 98, 100–102; and comforting 114–115; comforting and warming up by 8; connecting through 38; as coping strategy 80; and creative approach 55; exploration through 30; and integrative approach 71, 73–74, 80, 84–87, 91; between languages 15, 30; between materials 15; and perfectionism 110–111; between pretend world and the present moment 75–76; and sand tray 57, 69–61, 63; and sensory materials 19; through space 15; and trust 93–96; visual expression of 159
Mullin, J. 150
multisensory interventions 52, 57, 95, 142, 166, 174
Mundy, P. 45
music 8, 13–14, 93–94, 104, 163–168; and adolescents 137–138; and empathy 120; and engagement of children in therapy 15, 16, 19–20; and feelings 36, 38–41; instruments 8, 14–15, 19–20, 22, 36, 40–41, 75, 80, 83, 93, 98, 116, 164; in integrative approach 83–84, 91; and strong image 29, 32
mutual empathy 119

Nader-Grosbois, N. 117
natural interest, of children 57–59, 63
natural materials 105–106, 112–113, 132, 135
nature 8, 9, 33, 40, 47, 51–52, 54–55, 59–60, 91–92, 101–102, 104, 125, 129, 133–135, 144, 146, 149, 151
neurodiversity 45, 54
neurological 4, 17, 45, 53, 62, 85–88, 93, 129, 164, 167
neurological approach 95
neurological aspects of autism 86
neurological challenges 167
neurological integration 88–90
new learning 16, 23–24, 33, 88, 174
nightmares 66, 135
nondirective play therapy 75, 82
nonverbal communication 5, 101, 106, 142, 154–155, 167; engagement of children in therapy 15–16, 24, 27; in integrative approach 71, 73, 89, 91; and strong image 29, 35

occupational therapy 53, 168
Ohrt, J. H. 86
open ended (approaches in therapy) 39, 70, 74–76, 112, 137, 145, 167, 171
openness 80, 88
Orbach, N. 28, 146
Osborne, N. 154
overconnectivity, 51
own world, creation of 62, 69

painting 8, 12–15, 69, 169, 171–172; apps 149; and autism spectrum and continuum 142–143, 145, 147–149, 151, 153–154, 159–162; and clay 101–104; and empathy 120, 130–132, 140; engagement of children in therapy 17, 21–22, 24, 26; and feelings 37–39, 44; in integrative approach 70, 77, 81; and perfectionism 112; and trust 94–95, 97
parachutes 87

parent and child, joint sessions with 121–122, 154
parents 55, 121, 154–155, 164
parents, relationships of 51–52
Park, Clara 21
Park, Jessica 21
Penfold, L. 33
perceptual/affective level 155–158
perceptual experience 156
perfectionism 16, 24–27, 34, 72, 90, 108–110, 112, 134
Perry, D. 39
personal narrative 31, 90
perspective 4, 9, 11, 13, 20, 26, 45–46, 51, 53, 62, 71, 81, 94, 109, 117–118, 135, 138, 155–156, 159, 174
pervasive developmental disorder 49, 52, 54
Pfeifer, L. I. 75
phototherapy 121
physical movement in images 94
physical space 93–94
physical therapy 164, 168
physical uncomfortableness 84–85
Picasso 160
pillows 110, 139
planning sessions 84
play 1, 4–6, 8–9, 11–20, 22–23, 26–34, 36–44, 46, 57, 59–64, 67–78, 80–84, 86–87, 89, 91–94, 96, 100, 102–116, 118, 120, 123, 125–127, 129–130, 132–133, 135, 137, 143–145, 148, 156, 158, 171–174
playfulness 94
play therapy 1, 5, 14, 27, 38, 71, 73–75, 81–82, 84, 86
Pliske, M. 84
Porges, S. 49, 71, 85, 88, 94–95, 165
portraits creation 17, 73, 90, 147–148, 153
potential versus need 29
preferred images, of children 158
pretending 73, 113
pretend play 75–76, 94, 100, 113
prisms 9, 174
Prizant, B. 6, 16, 36, 47, 52–53, 81, 86–88, 90, 94, 143–144
processes 4, 8, 16, 21–23, 27–28, 33, 39, 47, 51, 57, 71, 74, 81, 87, 89, 91, 101, 105–106, 118, 132–134, 142–144, 148, 150, 153–154, 171, 174
Proulx, L. 142

psychotherapy 4–5, 53
puppets 14, 63, 110, 113–114, 137, 172; engagement of children in therapy 15, 19; and feelings 36, 41; in integrative approach 73–75, 82, 89

rapport building 71, 86
Ray, D. 73
reciprocal play 31, 34
reciprocal relationships 52, 68, 78
reciprocity 30, 39, 80
Regensburg, E. 20
Reggio Emilia Italy 15, 28–29, 31–33, 100
relational perspective of art 20
relationships 1, 4, 11, 14–15, 17, 20–21, 23–24, 28, 31, 33, 42, 51, 55, 62, 68, 70, 72–73, 76, 81, 83, 86–88, 91, 93–94, 97–98, 101, 103–104, 106, 111–112, 115–116, 132, 135, 138, 142, 145–146, 150–152, 154, 161, 164
relaxation 8, 13–14, 36, 142–143, 151, 158, 163, 173; and adolescents 129–130, 137; engagement of children in therapy 19, 24, 26; in integrative approach 75, 77, 82, 84, 86, 92; and perfectionism 108, 110–111, 113, 115; and sand tray 60, 62, 66; and trust 94
repetitive behaviors 53, 62, 87, 130, 154, 156
repetitive motions 94
repetitive play or imagery 34, 174
"rescuing" process 24–26
responsive materials 8, 39, 91, 98, 143, 149, 151
responsiveness 75, 82, 86
Rhyne, J. 90
rhythms 14, 24, 94, 96, 164, 167–168; autism spectrum and continuum 142, 149–151, 154, 159; and breathing 85; and feelings 36–37, 39–40; in integrative approach 80, 85, 87, 91; and perfectionism 113; and adolescents 129, 133; and sand 60–61; and strong image 31
Richardson, J. 97
Riley-Hall, E. 48
Rimland, M. 51–52, 55
Rinaldi, C. 29–31
Robbins, A. 150
Ross, M. 159

Rubin, J. 14, 20.22, 24, 96, 145
rules, of play 109, 113, 156
rumbling 115–116
Russo, F. A. 166–167

safe relationship 94
safe space 14, 87, 94, 120
safety, sense of 34, 66–67, 70–71, 73, 84, 91, 93–94, 108, 168
sand/sand tray 1, 9–12, 17–18, 68–69, 109, 112–113, 171; and adolescents 129, 132–133; autism spectrum and continuum 153, 156, 158; characters/figures of 36–38, 63–64, 66–68, 73, 82–83, 125–127, 133, 171, 173; and connection with nature 91–92; and creation/world building 57–62, 67–68, 70, 78, 104–106, 135, 173–174; and empathy 123–124; and exploration of feelings 43, 137–138, 176; and feelings 36–38, 41–43; and freedom 38, 63; in integrative approach 71, 73; kinaesthetic process 62; playing in the sand, purpose of 57–63; Sandtray/Worldplay 1, 9, 11–13, 63, 113–114; sensations and perceptions 38–39, 57, 62; and storytelling 8, 38, 41–42, 63, 76
satisfaction in learning, sense of 151
scaffolding 23, 27, 33–34, 81, 156
scarves 12, 36, 40, 70, 75, 87, 135
SCERTS model 14n1, 144
Schadler, G. 27, 71
Schuler, A. 81
Schweizer, C. 143
scribbling/scribble chase 154
self-awareness 6–7, 19, 27–28, 70, 85, 88, 129, 150, 163, 168
self-doubt 78
self-efficacy 6, 27–28, 59, 63, 70, 130, 132
self-exploration 140
self-expression 6–7, 15, 168
self-regulation 23–24, 33, 37, 52, 75, 82, 84, 86, 95–96, 109, 172, 174
self-soothing behaviors 16, 85, 96, 111
senses 4–5, 31, 37, 44, 46, 70, 78, 80, 117, 143, 172, 174–176; and AMT 166; and clay 100–103, 105; and energy 159; and natural materials 112; regulation through 151; and sand 38, 57–60, 62, 105, 112

sensory challenges 4, 73, 94, 130, 149–151, 164; addressing 46, 93; of high functioning autistic people 50; impact of 55, 93; and yoga 85–86
sensory comfort 95, 118–120
sensory experiences 80, 95, 98, 142, 152, 160
sensory exploration 133, 160
sensory imbalances 78
sensory materials 19, 24, 72, 87, 98, 112, 139–140, 147, 154, 159, 171
sensory-motor integrative experience 39
sensory needs 87, 143, 149
sensory preferences 8, 112, 132, 143–144, 155–156
sensory profiles 1, 23, 33, 146, 164
sensory responses 59–62, 144–146; and process and perception of individuals 146; regulation of 16, 22–23
sensory sensitivities 52, 93, 143–144, 148
sensory stimulation 102, 144, 151
sensory system 51–52
Shanker, S. 27
Sharma, S. 160
Sheffer, E. 54
Shore, S. 14, 19–20, 22, 39–40, 46–47, 105
Sibley, L. 150
Siegel, D. 8, 31, 87–88, 91, 95, 167
Silberman, S. 51, 53
social action 32–33
social anxiety 53
social cognition, lack of 53
social communication 4–5, 16, 22–23, 144–145, 172
social deficit 53
social interaction 31, 46, 81
social responsiveness 75, 82
social settings comfort 13
sounds 15, 93, 119
space 87, 112; and clay figures 100, 102; movements through 15; neutrally instantiated we-centric space 119; physical 93–94; safe 14, 87, 94, 120; shared 22–23, 144; therapeutic 14–15, 60, 84, 104, 120, 140
special interests, connecting with 1, 8, 18–19, 30, 41–44, 47, 53, 81, 120–122
specialness 73
special rights, child with 29–30

spectrum 6, 31, 34, 45–50, 52–56, 86–88, 93–95, 146–147, 150
speech therapy 15, 53, 74, 164, 167
Stagnitti, K. 75
Steele, W. 84, 87
Stern, D. 118
stick puppets 89
stories 6, 11, 17, 31–32, 34, 36, 39–44, 57, 61, 64, 66, 90, 101, 106, 108, 118, 121, 130, 148, 158, 166–167, 172, 174
storytelling 30–32, 36, 103, 106, 155; and sand/sand tray 8, 38, 41–42, 63, 76; sense of 90; sharing of 80; verbal story 37, 61–62, 67–68, 76
strengths, focusing on 30–31, 70
stress 9, 46, 48, 80, 85–86, 104, 111, 119, 129–130, 145, 174
stress and stressors 46, 73, 85, 87, 129
stress balls 174
stretch cloths 76, 87
strong image of children 5, 11, 22, 28–35, 132, 160
structure (in therapy) 6, 30, 35, 49, 71–72, 75, 81, 83, 101, 105, 120, 146, 164, 166, 174
symbolic behavior/communication 34, 44, 57, 60, 63, 100, 144, 155, 158; engagement of children in therapy 16–17, 22–23, 27; in integrative approach 71, 73; and trust 95–96
symbolic play 44, 63
symbols 27, 59, 63, 69, 145

talk therapy *see* psychotherapy
Tammet, Daniel 38–39
therapeutic goals 5–6, 16, 36, 46, 71, 73, 75
therapeutic riding 168
therapeutic space 14–15, 60, 84, 104, 120, 140
third eye 22, 96
"third hand" support 24–27, 34, 66, 101, 156
three-dimensional medium 96, 100–101, 146, 148; *see also* clay
timetable 81
Tolleson Robles, M. 160–162
top-down 152–153
Tortora, S. 39, 119
Traditional Chinese Medicine, perspective on therapists 46–47

transactional support 34, 144–145
transformation 100, 131, 145
trauma 86
Treffert, D. 147
Trevarthen, C. 96
trust 5, 20, 71, 86, 90, 93–97, 146

Underconnectivity 51

Van Lith, T. 75, 81, 152–153
Vecchi, V. 101, 106, 145, 150
verbal communication 14, 64, 142, 144, 158, 167; engagement of children in therapy 16, 24, 26–27; in integrative approach 70, 87; and strong image 30, 34–35
verbal languages 15, 39, 62–63, 106
verbal story 37, 61–62, 67–68, 76
virtual tele-play 148
visual experience, art making as 145
visual expression 31, 39, 70, 91, 142, 159
visual languages 15–16, 30, 106, 158
Vygotsky, L. 23, 33–34, 118

Wadeson, H. 146
Walker, N. 45–46, 53
Weiser, J. 121
Werner, H. 159–161
Wetherby, A. M. 16, 34, 144
Wheelwright, S. 117
Whitehouse, A. 50
Wieder, S. 55, 63, 73
Wilkerson, L. 132
Wilkinson, R. 131
Williams, D. 21
Wing, L. 53–54
Winnicott, D. 29, 70
Wolfberg, P. 22, 34, 81, 113
world building, and sand tray 57
World Health Organization (WHO) 50
worries 6–7, 46, 81–82, 98, 113–115, 118, 126, 130, 137

xylophone 8, 14, 19, 22, 40–41, 83, 93, 98

yoga 84–86, 111

Zeldovich, L. 51
zone of proximal development 33

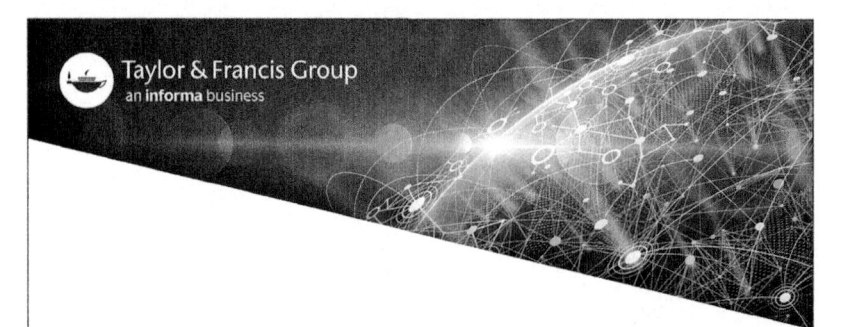

Printed in Great Britain
by Amazon